# TIBETAN SECRETS

## 5 STEPS TO UNLIMITED ENERGY AND RESTORED HEALTH

*3rd Edition*

*by Mary Solomon*

# © Copyright 2015-Mary Solomon All rights reserved.

In no way is it legal to reproduce, duplicate, or transmit any part of this document in either electronic means or in printed format. Recording of this publication is strictly prohibited and any storage of this document is not allowed unless with written permission from the publisher. All rights reserved.

The information provided herein is stated to be truthful and consistent, in that any liability, in terms of inattention or otherwise, by any usage or abuse of any policies, processes, or directions contained within is the solitary and utter responsibility of the recipient reader. Under no circumstances will any legal responsibility or blame be held against the publisher for any reparation, damages, or monetary loss due to the information herein, either directly or indirectly.
Respective authors own all copyrights not held by the publisher.

Legal Notice:
This book is copyright protected. This is only for personal use. You cannot amend, distribute, sell, use, quote or paraphrase any part or the content within this book without the consent of the author or copyright owner. Legal action will be pursued if this is breached.

Disclaimer Notice:
Please note the information contained within this document is for educational and entertainment purposes only. Every attempt has been made to provide accurate, up to date and reliable complete information. No warranties of any kind are

expressed or implied. Readers acknowledge that the author is not engaging in the rendering of legal, financial or professional advice.

By reading this document, the reader agrees that under no circumstances are we responsible for any losses, direct or indirect, which are incurred as a result of the use of information contained within this document, including, but not limited to, —errors, omissions, or inaccuracies.

# Table of Contents

TIBETAN SECRETS

*5 STEPS TO UNLIMITED ENERGY AND RESTORED HEALTH*

THE HISTORY OF THE FIVE TIBETAN RITES

PRACTICAL ADVANTAGES OF THE FIVE TIBETAN RITES

THE FIVE TIBETAN RITES OF REJUVENATION

BENEFITS OF THE FIVE TIBETAN RITES

THE SCIENCE BEHIND THE BENEFITS

THE SIXTH RITE

THE ESSENCE OF THE SIXTH RITE:

MODIFICATION OF THE FIVE TIBETAN RITES

TIBETAN MEDICINE

THE FLOW OF TIBETAN MEDICINE

CAUSES OF DISEASES ACCORDING TO TIBETAN MEDICINE

DIAGNOSIS IN TIBETAN MEDICINE

COMPONENTS OF TIBETAN MEDICINE

TREATMENT IN TIBETAN MEDICINE

THE TIBETAN MASSAGE

TIBETAN MEDICINE AND PHYSICAL DECAY

HOW TO DEAL WITH DISEASES

CHAKRAS EXPLAINED

HUMAN AURA

FAQS ON THE TOPIC

MINDFULNESS AND THE 5 RITES

**THE IMPORTANCE OF MEDITATION AND ITS TYPES**

**YOGA POSES THAT COMPLEMENT THE 5 TIBETAN RITES**

**TIBETAN SINGING BOWLS**

**IMPORTANT NATURAL SUPPLEMENTS THAT FIGHT INFLAMMATION**

**THE 5 RITES AND FOOD RULES**

**HOW TO MAKE IT A HABIT**

**CONCLUSION**

# Introduction

Imagine, just for a moment – visualize the Himalayas – mighty, majestic, snow clad.... and a feeling of tranquility and bliss enveloping us. We all yearn to go there and experience the serenity, the peace that is a part of this beautiful place. Someday (we make a mental promise to ourselves).... someday we will take a break from our hectic schedules and spend some time amidst the beauty of the Himalayas and discover our inner selves. No family to take care of, no demands to be met, no deadlines – just one resolute soul determined to spend some time experiencing bliss, joy, silence and solitude amidst nature.

Sounds like a farfetched dream and we briskly shake our heads as reality jolts us back to earth and we go about the business of leading our lives. Is this state of mind really so elusive? Can we not experience bliss, stillness of mind and a calm and composed outlook in our daily lives? Most of us have heard about yoga and meditation. We know someone who practices it regularly and are fully aware of all the health benefits of yoga. But we feel it is too idealistic and very impractical to incorporate it into our daily schedules, or we need to learn it from a yoga practitioner or join a class. Exercising in the gym, too, requires time and money. So we just keep postponing the inevitable.

Until a day arrives, when we lose your temper for no concrete reason, or those aches and pains have developed into acute problems and we feel we have reached our physical, mental and emotional threshold. We decide that the least we can do is make a beginning somewhere. We weigh the pros and cons of our particular situation and want to go in for something which is not time consuming, yet gives us all the benefits of exercising. We look for ways and means of doing something, which will not cost us a lot of money. And with a little research, we will realize that the Tibetan rites meet all of our requirements completely.

The Tibetan Rites has been practiced for over 2000 years. These five simple steps have proven to slow the aging process, help produce and restore energy and lead to restored health. These five simple steps can change your life.

# The History Of The Five Tibetan Rites

There is an interesting story behind the Tibetan rites: 2500 years ago, a boy called Peter Kelder is believed to have lived in the mid – west United States. Some people believe that he was an adopted child and left home as a teenager. During his travels, Peter met a retired British army colonel named Colonel Bradford, in Southern California. Colonel Bradford narrated his traveling experiences to Kelder.

When the Colonel was posted in India, the natives told him about a group of lamas who seemed to have discovered the 'fountain of youth'. They told him that old, stooped men who walked with the support of a cane were transformed into healthy, strong and virile men who could walk without any support after their stay in the lamasery.

Colonel Bradford searched for the lamasery after his retirement and lived with these Tibetan monks/lamas. These Tibetan monks taught him the five Tibetan rites or exercises. They are similar to the yoga postures practiced widely in India, but the Tibetan rites emphasize movements, whereas the yoga postures are mainly static.

The Lamas explained the concept of the seven chakras or psychic vortexes to the Colonel. These chakras are actually spinning electromagnetic fields of different colors and fill us with energy as they spin. These chakras are located above the major endocrine glands of the body. Enough evidence has been found to prove that the hormones produced from these endocrine glands regulate the aging process.

These chakras should ideally be spinning in synchronization at top speed. But stress, old age, faulty diet, faulty eating habits, improper food combinations, etc. cause these chakras to spin at a slower pace.

Practicing these five simple movements boosts the spin rate of these chakras, which normalizes the hormonal imbalances of the body resulting in improved health and longevity. It makes the person feel energetic and fills him with a sense of vitality and well being.

Practicing the five Tibetan rites daily stimulates all the seven chakras and makes them spin rapidly at the same rate. When one of these chakras is blocked, the natural spin rate slows down, thereby blocking the flow of vital life energy or prana. When the circulation of this life energy is blocked, illness, stress, aging, pain, etc. is experienced.

We will look at all the chakras in detail in a future chapter and tell you how you can fix each if there is a lot of blockage in them. This is only to help you perform the exercises with ease and add leverage to your workouts.

Colonel Bradford was also taught a sixth rite. But the Lamas recommend this rite only for those who are willing to practice celibacy and live a chaste life that is free from all forms of temptations, both physical and mental in nature.

Peter Kelder first publicized these Tibetan rites in 1939, in a 32-pages booklet titled, "The Eye of Revelation". In this booklet, Kelder discusses his interaction with Colonel Bradford, who gives simple, precise, detailed instructions on how the Tibetan rites need to be practiced.

The emphasis on following a particular breathing pattern is not clearly implied in the original booklet. Later editions by other people recommend following a particular breathing pattern for better results and also have a word of caution for people with certain and specific health conditions or illnesses.

# Practical Advantages Of The Five Tibetan Rites

- It requires a minimum of only 10 minutes and a maximum of twenty minutes of our time. The benefits are really worth the time.

- It doesn't cost any money.

- These movements are easy to understand and learn. We do not need an expert to guide us.

- The best part is – we can practice these movements without stepping out of our homes, but also if we are traveling.

- We can reap the benefits of the Tibetan rites by doing it indoors, regardless of the weather conditions outside.

- The Tibetan rites do not require any special equipment.

- All we need to do is spread a rug or blanket or towel on the floor.

- We need just enough space to lie down and move our arms and legs.

- These Tibetan rites can be practiced at any time of the day or evening. (The benefits are enhanced if the rites are performed at daybreak and at sunset - but we can really do them whenever it is convenient for us).

## Recommandations For Beginners

- Avoid doing these exercises on a full stomach.

- Wear loose, comfortable clothes.

- It is advisable to do them in a well-ventilated area (outdoors if possible – but not in the hot sun).

- Start these exercises at a slow pace initially.

- Follow the order of the exercises.

- Initially start by performing each Tibetan rite 3 times in one day.

- Listen to your body. Avoid straining your body.

- Refrain from holding on to a position if you feel any pain or think that you may injure yourself.

- You may feel a little sore initially, but by the next day you will be fine.

- After a week's interval, increase the number of repetitions for each rite to 5.

- Keep adding 2 repetitions per week till you reach 21 repetitions per day.

- Once your body has gained strength and endurance, it will take you less than 20 minutes in all to do all the 21 repetitions for each rite.

- Improve the speed with which each exercise has to be performed gradually.

- It is more important to do the exercises correctly than to do them quickly, but incorrectly.

- Ensure that you follow the breathing pattern correctly.

- Holding your breath during the exercises or improper breathing patterns may lead to tiredness or light-headedness.

- Ensure that you take at least three cleansing breaths after each exercise.

- The essence of the healing powers of the five Tibetan rites lies in holding the position for at least 2 or 3 seconds.

- Try to do these exercises at least five times in a week.

- It is better to do fewer repetitions of all the exercises every day than postponing it to another day when you have time for the entire regimen.

- Each rite should be repeated to a maximum of 21 times only.

- Avoid over doing these exercises.

- These rites are essentially for restoring the energy flow of our body, which indirectly benefits us in various ways.

- If you want to do more than 21 repetitions, adding another session later on during the day can prove to be beneficial.

- Refrain from doing these rites in the late evening or just before you go to bed.

- The 5 Tibetan rites should ideally be done after your morning shower.

- If the 5 Tibetan rites are done correctly, you should not perspire at all.

- Showering after doing the 5 Tibetan rites will prove to be ineffective as water dissipates all the prana/life energy that the exercises have built up in the body.

- It is advisable to perform these 5 Tibetan exercises in the early morning as they boost the metabolism of the body for the rest of the day and burn more body fat.

These rites will fill you up with energy that lasts for hours. While this is a great way to start the day, performing these rites in the late evening will result in building up a lot of energy for hours and we may find it difficult to fall asleep at night.

# The Five Tibetan Rites of Rejuvenation

The exercises are physical demanding, but supply the body with energy for hours. The Tibetans feel that these physical movements are not exercises and prefer to call them rites. So we will use the term the five Tibetan rites throughout this book.

## *The First Rite/ Clock-Wise Spin*

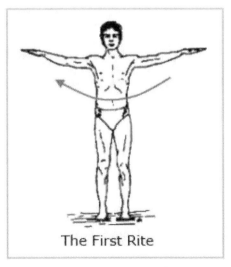

- Stand straight keeping your spinal cord erect.

- Stretch your arms ensuring that they are straight and parallel to the floor.

- Your palms must be facing downwards with the fingers close together.

- Inhale deeply through your nose during the first spin

- Assuming that the floor had a clock on it, start spinning around very slowly in the clockwise direction until you complete 3 spins initially.

- Ensure that you are spinning around on the same spot.

- Exhale deeply through the mouth.

- After each cycle of 3 spins, place your hands on your hips with your feet apart.

- Breathe naturally.

- Begin with three spins and slowly work up to 21 repetitions.

- Look at a particular point steadily if you are feeling dizzy.

- Take two slow deep breaths after you finish this rite while you feel the sensations in your body.

- Relax for a few seconds before you start the second rite.

- Begin with three and gradually work your way up to 21 repetitions.

## *Benefits:*

- Refreshes and revitalizes the body. The spinning will help your balance and the alignment will improve. There are many people whose balance will be off and they will not be able to even walk in a straight line. They will start to swagger and not have the capacity to walk from point A to point B in a straight line. So just by performing this first rite, it will be possible for the person to balance himself or herself.

- Enhances the coordination between your eye and hand. This means that you will be able to see something and act on it faster. So you can see something once and then reach for it without having to see it through. So it is best to perform this rite if you have a problem with this type of coordination.

- Harmonizes the spin rates of all the chakras. We know how important all the chakras in the body are. They rotate to help the body remain healthy. It is possible for the person to have umpteen healthy only if their chakras are spinning properly. When you spin around, the chakras will spin accordingly. So it is best to spin clock wise, which is the direction in which the chakras spin. There are theories, which claim turning anti clockwise helps the body. But this might not be correct and the best way to spin is to turn clockwise.

- It is also possible for you to beat the blues with this movement. This means that your mental make up will improve when you turn around. The turning around will ensure that you are having fun and it is increasing the release of dopamine. So if you are feeling low, then the best thing to do is spin around. You will feel an instant mood lift. This is especially important to take up if you are feeling angered or stressed as well. If you think someone is annoying you, then take his or her leave and start spinning around! You will only feel better about it.

- In the Sufi culture, they turn around and look upwards. This helps them connect better spiritually and calm down. So you will experience the same and feel a higher level of spirituality.

- Physically speaking, the fat in your mid riff area as well as your arms will start to reduce and you will also feel lighter as the fat in your lower back will start to melt away.

These are just some of the benefits of the first rite and are not limited to just these. As and when you practice the rites, you will be acquainted with the others.

## *The Second Rite/ Raised Legs*

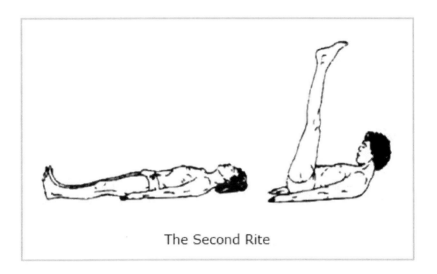

The Second Rite

- Lie down flat on the mat placed on the floor, keeping your face upwards.

- Ensure that your arms are straight and parallel to your body.

- Let the palms touch the mat and ensure that are fingers are close together.

- Take a deep breath through your nose.

- Slowly, lift your head away from the floor and bring it against your chest.

- Ensure that the chin touches the chest.

- Simultaneously, lift your legs away from the floor while keeping them straight (No bending at the knees.)

- Lift your legs till they are at 90 degrees to your body.

- Try to move the legs further (bending at the hips, not the knees) and bring them towards your head, but do not let the knees bend.

- Gradually, lower the head and the legs to the floor.

- Let the muscles relax as you exhale through the mouth

- Inhale and exhale deeply twice after you complete each exercise.

- Take two deep breaths after you finish this rite and feel the sensations in your body.

- Relax for a few seconds before you start the third rite.

- Begin with three and gradually work your way up to 21 repetitions.

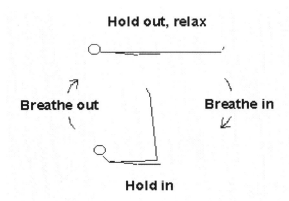

## Benefits:

- Improves clarity of mind and instills a sense of calmness and peace. This is extremely important. In this day and age where everything is chaotic, it is important that you find a peace of mind and remain calm in even the harshest of situations. If you remain distracted by the chaos, then you will not be able to make quick and meaningful decisions. So by taking up this exercise, you will calm down and have the chance to think straight.

- You will also find that you are able to digest food faster and in a proper way. Your rate of metabolism will increase and the food that you take in will be digested faster. There is a similar pose in yoga, which is adopted to eliminate flatulence from your body. So if you are the type that eats all the wrong food types and feels bloated all the time, then it is best to take up this exercise and eliminate the build up of gas in your body. You will see that your bloated feeling has disappeared and you are feeling lighter. Do this the next day after you have eaten something that is gastric, such as peanuts and potatoes.

- Strengthens and tones the hips, lower back, legs and neck. The hips are an issue for many women. They will wish for the fat in their hips to disappear. The best way to make that possible is by performing this exercise. You can also strengthen the muscles in your lower back and neck. If you are having a lot of problem in the muscles in your neck owing to staring at a computer screen, then it is best to perform this exercise. You will find that there is no pain in your neck and your lower back.

- As the movement calls for your neck to be pulled up and your legs to be pulled in, you will have the chance to tone the muscles in your stomach. If you are having a problem in starting an exercise routine, then it is best to take up this form of exercise. It will help you get accustomed to the routine. It will fill you up with enthusiasm and help you take up other forms of exercise.

Your posture will improve when you take up this exercise. There are many people who will display a little stoop when they walk and the best solution for this is to take up this form of exercise.

## *The Third Rite/Back Bend On Knees*

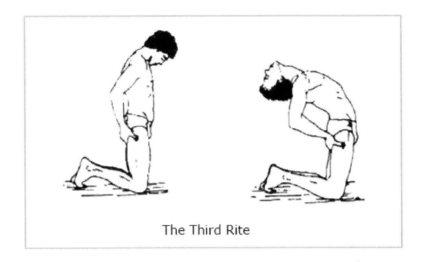

The Third Rite

- Kneel down on the mat, which is placed on the floor, knees slightly apart, toes curled, keeping your spinal cord straight.
- Place your hands against your thigh muscles.
- Bring the head and neck forward to make it touch the chest.

- Ensure that the chin touches the chest.
- Take a deep breath through your nose.
- Fill your lungs completely with air.
- Take your head and neck backwards now, arching the spine.

- As your shoulder blades come together, try to bend the head and the neck backwards as far as you comfortably can.

- You can feel your lower spine relaxing.

- Support your arms and hands by placing them against the thighs as you bend backwards.

- Avoid bending beyond the waist level.

- Do not strain yourself unduly.

- Return to the original position of your chin touching your chest

- Breathe out through the mouth.

- Your lungs should be thoroughly empty when you reach the original position.

- Take two deep cleansing breaths between each repetition.

- Take two deep breaths after you finish this rite and feel the sensations in your body.

- Relax for a few seconds before you start the fourth rite.

- As with the other rites, start with three and work your way up to 21 repetitions.

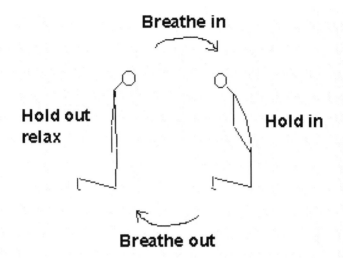

Benefits:

- Makes the body flexible. Having a stiff body is something that anybody would hate. Imagine how it would feel to walk around in a stiff posture where you have to turn around half your body just to look to your side. It will feel extremely horrible. So to fix this issue and have a flexible body, you need to perform this rite. You will also have the chance to bend down and pick up something with ease and save yourself a lot of embarrassment. It will also be possible for you to play with your children and keep up with them physically.

- Enhances receptivity of the mind. This means that you can remain alert and interpret something fast enough. The human mind is capable of analyzing something with ease and interpreting it with equal ease. But if there are a lot of distractions, then the mind will not be able to process something fast enough. This might be because of both mental and physical stimulus. In such a situation, the person might feel extremely distracted and in need of better concentration. But just by performing this exercise, it is possible for your mind to be better receptive to information and be ready with an answer within a few minutes of receiving the information.

- Boosts the energy flow to the heart chakra. The heart chakra is located right next to the heart and when you bend backwards your chest completely stretches out. Opening up this chakra will make you an emotional person and help you connect with others in a better way. Your relationships will also improve and you and your spouse will have a better-married life. The heart chakra also deals with being disappointed by others out of having high emotional expectations. By performing this exercise, you will become a bit more practical and not fall for others emotionally easily.

- Gives relief from muscle tension. Many people have spasms in their back owing to maintaining the same posture for long. But just by performing these exercises, it is possible for you to avail instant relief from all your back problems. It will be difficult for you to get up from your chair in office sometimes owing to maintaining a stiff back. But this problem can be effectively dealt with by performing this exercise. But don't think of it as a means to an end. You will not be able to beat the occurrence of the spasm and only have the chance to reduce the occurrence of the spasm. You will also be able to get up from your seat fast enough.

- Stretches the muscles. Muscles are an important part of your body. They will cut out the fat in your body and make sure that you remain lean. If you take up cardio exercises, then there is always the danger of burning away the essential muscles. But this problem can be remedied by performing this activity. Just spend some time to perform the 5 rites and you will realize how beneficial it really is for your body.

- Lengthens and tones the spine. The spine is extremely important for all human beings. It supports your back and gives you a proper figure. Those who assume the wrong posture will end up affecting their spine. This will mean that their back is strained and they are not able to function properly. So the best remedy to this problem is to perform this rite. Get into this position and you feel rejuvenated. You will feel that all your pain has vanished and your position has changed for the better.

## *The Fourth Rite/Table top*

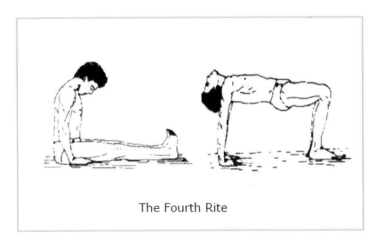

The Fourth Rite

- Sit straight up on the mat and keep your legs outstretched in front of you.

- Ensure that your feet are around 12 inches apart.

- Let your palms rest on the mat, fingers together, near your buttocks.

- Bring your chin forward so that it rests against the chest.

- Take a deep breath through your nose.

- Now, take your head backwards fully.

- Simultaneously, raise your buttocks and bend your knees as raise your body.

- The weight of your body will automatically shift to your arms.

- Using your arms for support, continue to raise your buttocks until your midsection and thighs are straight and parallel to the floor.

- Allow your head to arch backwards as much as you possibly can.

- Now, your body will be supported with your arms and lower legs only.

- Hold your breath as you feel the tension in every muscle of the body.

- Breathe out completely through your mouth as you lower your body to the floor.

- Return to the original sitting position allowing your chin to touch your chest.

- Inhale and exhale deeply twice as you rest between repetitions.

- Take two deep breaths and feel the sensations in your body.

- Relax for a few seconds before you start the fifth rite.

- Begin with three and gradually work your way up to 21 repetitions.

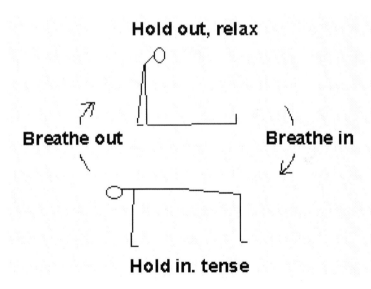

Benefits:

•       Stimulates the hormonal glands. The hormones are extremely important for the body. If you have your hormones mixed up then your body will suffer. There are many hormonal glands in the body and each one has a specific function in the body. If these glands won't function properly then you will start to feel stressed out and also have other problems such as those that affect your reproductive system. So it is best to have all your hormones in check. It is observed that instead of relying on medicines to help regularize your hormones, the best way to fix them is by performing physical activities. This posture is great to get all your hormones in shape and get them to function properly. It is for all those that are feeling stressed and want to get over it.

•       Enhances the stability and balance of the entire body. It is important to balance the stability of the body. If you have instability in your body, then you will wobbly. So the best way to fix this issue is by performing this exercise. Just get into this posture for a month or two and you will see the difference that it has on your posture. Continue with it and don't give up. Remain within your comfort zone and don't try to over do it as that might cause a spasm or a muscle pull. That might cause you to stop for some time and lower your confidence in these exercises.

•       Improves the functioning of the circulatory and lymphatic systems. Blood is very important for the body. It not only helps in carrying out fresh oxygen to the different parts of the body but also assists in eliminating the waste from the body. So it is important to have your blood in constant circulation. Many times, the circulation slows down owing to the presence of toxins in the blood. So the best thing to do is to perform this pose and eliminate the toxins from blood. It is possible to do so by getting into positions that will help cleanse the blood. It will also help circulate the blood in all the parts of the body.

- Strengthens the wrists, arms, shoulders and lower body. This pose will help in strengthening your wrists and shoulders, which are generally ignored. Many people do not perform exercises that help their arms and hands. So it is important perform exercises that affect these areas. By performing these exercises you will strengthen your shoulders and wrists. If after a very long time you have lifted something heavy, then you will suddenly feel a sharp pain shoot up and you might have to visit the doctor for the pain to subside. This is because you are not accustomed to it. So the best thing to do to protect your arms and wrist is to perform this exercise regularly and strengthen your arms to help them lift heavy things.

## The Fifth Rite/ Pendulum

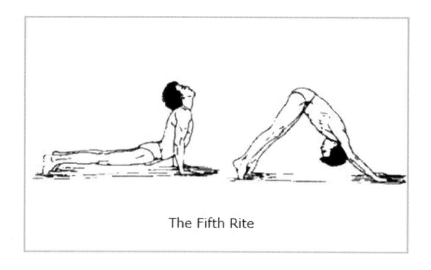

The Fifth Rite

- Position your body such that if faces downwards towards the floor.

- Ensure that your hands and feet are always straight while performing this movement.

- Breathe in deeply through your nose.

- Flexing your toes and using your arms for support, raise your body away from the floor as your arch your spine (like push- ups).

- Keep your head straight/Look directly in front of you.

- Slowly bend your head backwards.

- Except your curled toes and your arms, no part of your body should be touching the ground.

- Raise your hips gradually, push your buttocks up into the air and lift the entire body to form an inverted V shape.

- Ensure that your legs and arms are straight.

- Bring the head forward ensuring that the chin touches the chest.

- Try to make the soles of your feet touch the floor completely.

- Breathe out slowly as you lower your body.

- Return to the original position slowly (arms supporting your weight and head held backwards.

- Take two cleansing breaths between each movement.

- Begin with 3 and gradually work your way up to 21 repetitions.

- Take two deep breaths and feel the sensations in your body.

- Lie down flat on the mat on your stomach with your arms stretched out in front of you, head on one side and your eyes closed.

- Relax completely and allow your heartbeats and breathing to return to normal.

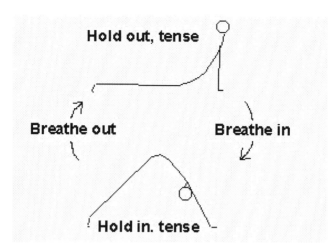

Benefits:

- Energizes the body. It is important to energize your body from time to time. Given the amount of work we do these days, it is important for the body to remain with a lot of energy. Performing this posture can do this. Don't expect results over night though. If you do it for a month, then you will see results the next month and so on. Don't compare yourself with another person as the exercises work differently for everyone. Don't over do it just because you want to end up with a lot of energy. Do how much ever is possible and more importantly, do it in the prescribed amount. You will feel more energetic and be left with a lot more energy than what you normally had before.

  - Gives us relief from fatigue and stress. If you are fatigued and just cannot stop feeling tired all the time, then you can perform this pose. Many times we will have a truckload of enthusiasm to do something but will not be able to perform the task. This is because your body will be extremely tired and not able to move a single muscle in your body without feeling tired. So in order to avoid such a situation, you can perform this exercise and increase your body's capacity to cope with physical demands. You won't have to make something wait just because you don't have the energy for it. It also assists in cutting down on stress as it is possible for the mind to control the body and make it feel tired even if the body by itself is not feeling tired. So you must work on both these levels to cut out the stress and fatigue from your body and feel energized.

- Enhances the flexibility of the body and makes almost every muscle of our body strong. You need to add in flexibility to your body in order to better perform the various routines in life. If you are flexible, then you can easily avoid all spasms and other such problems. You might have to go to office having a bad backache, which can easily be avoided by performing the 5 rites regularly. This posture, in particular, is great for the back and helps in stretching the spine and strengthening your back muscles, which are important for strength and stability.

- Motivates us to pursue this form of exercise regularly. This is extremely important. You have to remain strong for long and for that, you must exercises regularly. You cannot take it up for one month, see difference and stop. You must make it a regular activity and incorporate exercise into your regular routine. Make sure you add the 5 rites to your routine and all of them, not just any one of the exercises. Remain invested in them and reap the benefits of these rites to energize your body for life.

## What to do after you finish doing the five Tibetan rites:

- The 5 Tibetan rites can be performed as a standalone form of energizing yourself or...

- You can perform these exercises as a way of warming up for any other form of exercise.

- After you finish performing these exercises, walk around for a couple of minutes or do some light stretching exercises before you go about your daily activities.

- Some people prefer to meditate after performing the Tibetan Rites. This has proved to be an excellent way of enhancing the benefits of the five Tibetan rites.


## A word of caution:

- People suffering from high blood pressure and heart problems must do rite 4 and 5 very slowly and ensure that they keep their head above the level of the heart.

- People who are on drugs that cause dizziness or are suffering from health conditions like heart problems, arthritis of the spine, high blood pressure, vertigo, hyperthyroid, etc. should consult their physicians before they start doing these exercises.

- Overweight people should refrain from doing rite 4 and 5 till they have developed ample physical endurance and strength.

# Benefits Of The Five Tibetan Rites

When all the five exercises are repeated 21 times, the benefits are immense.

- Reduced stress: You'll feel calmer as a person and are able to deal with stressful situations coolly. This is one thing that most people complain about. Given the type of hectic life that we lead, we end up undertaking a lot of stress. So it is important to remain as calm, cool and collected as possible at all times and this can only be possible if you perform the Tibetan rites on a regular basis.

- Increased energy in the body and mind: The energy that you get from performing the five Tibetan rites lasts for hours and is unlike the caffeinated boost of energy which exhausts us after a short while. In fact, these drinks will do more bad than good to your body and so; it is best to perform these rites as a great replacement for these drinks. You can get up early in the morning and perform these rites the first thing in the morning and remain energetic all through the day.

- Enhanced feeling of calmness, mental focus and clarity of thought: We are able to retain our composure during stressful times and think clearly. Many people think they cannot think clearly given the amount of stress that they undertake. So the best way to deal with this is by performing the five rites first thing in the morning as opposed to indulging in any other form of activity including checking your phone!

- Increased physical strength: These rites energize us thereby we don't feel exhausted or fatigued by physical work. With the amount of travelling and working that we do, it is only obvious that we will feel a lack of energy. The best way to beat this feeling is to practice the 5 rites on a regular basis and allow it to affect us both physically and mentally.

- Sharper memory: Reduced stress has a positive impact on our retention power leading to better memory power. This will allow you to have better conversations with others and remember important things for longer.

- Enhanced oxygen consumption by the body: The body consumes more oxygen when we take deep breaths while performing the rites. You know how important oxygen is for the body and just by performing these rites; you will have the chance to increase the intake.

- Improved respiration: With the additional oxygen that our body gets, our respiratory system is able to function more effectively.

- Weight loss around midsection: Some people find it easier to lose weight after performing the five Tibetan rites because they crave healthier foods. Other people feel this is an excellent way of controlling their weight.

- Improves muscle strength: After performing the five Tibetans, you may see your muscles building up on your arms, hips, legs, stomach and back. It tones flabby arms and tightens the abdominal muscles.

- Strengthens the spine: These movements give us relief from chronic backache.

- Deep restful sleep: Some people experience dreamless sleep while others have more vivid dreams.

- Relief from arthritis: When the prana/life energy flows freely through the body, people suffering from arthritis get a lot of relief from their joint pains.

- Builds up the stamina, endurance and immunity of the body: We don't seem to get sick as frequently and don't fall prey to common colds as easily.

- Improves circulation of the blood.

- Improves the efficiency of the heart.

- Relaxes the nervous system: We no longer suffer from mood swings and these exercises make us feel more in control of our emotions.

- Enhanced potency/sexual performance.

- Restoration of hair.

- Anti aging – makes you look youthful.

- Improves bone mass.

- Decreased pain.

- Better digestion and elimination.

# The Science Behind The Benefits

A combination of the five Tibetan rites followed by a session of meditation enhances the benefits that we gain after we do the five Tibetan rites. Scientific studies have proved that meditation is beneficial to the human body.

- In the year 2005, the Dalai Lama was invited to the annual meeting of the Society for Neuroscience in Washington D.C. During his speech, this great Tibetan spiritual leader emphasized the similarity between the Buddhist teachings and neuroscience.

- According to neuroscience, meditation is actually a series of mental exercises, which gives us the necessary mental strength to control the working of our own brain. Sufficient evidence has been gathered to prove that meditation and exercise has immense direct and indirect benefits on our body.

- It is now an accepted fact that there are tangible and intangible forces that are constantly working within our bodies and minds. Regular deep meditation improves the electromagnetic rhythm of the neurons and they start vibrating rapidly in harmony. That is why meditation is said to improve mood and health.

# The Sixth Rite

In the booklet titled "The Eye of Revelation" that was published in 1939, Colonel Bradford reveals to his students the existence of a sixth rite that can be done if they want to gain super powerful benefits and experience mysticism.

Colonel Bradford mentions in this booklet that the benefits of these five Tibetan rites are immense, and make one appear younger and more energetic, but if a person yearns to be young in the truest sense of the world, then he should learn the sixth rite.

In order to learn the sixth rite they:

- Would have to perform 21 repetitions of the first five Tibetans properly and gain all its benefits.

- Would have to lead celibate lives.

It must be kept in mind; however, that the monks who taught Colonel Bradford the 5 Tibetan rites were all male and were spiritually inclined. Celibacy was something that they had always been practicing.

Celibacy is not a choice that many men would opt for and just doing 21 repetitions of the five Tibetan rites is enough to experience the immense benefits mentioned in the booklet.

This does not necessarily mean that the sixth rite is not worth practicing. Most people are content leading normal, healthy and meaningful lives and are satisfied with the benefits of the first five Tibetan rites.

Most people who really yearn to master the technique of the sixth rite either want to at least attempt it and experience its benefits or are interested in researching the traditional Tantric practices.

In the booklet, "The Eye of Revelation" Colonel Bradford offers a word of caution for people who are keen on learning the sixth rite. He says:

"It is mandatory that a man be full of masculine virility in order to perform the sixth rite. He needs to transmute the procreative energy and for this to happen he needs be virile. It is impossible for an impotent man or a man with little virility to do the sixth rite. If he attempts to do so, it will have disastrous consequences, which may end up harming him thus leading to discouragement.

If he is really keen on mastering the sixth rite, he should first practice the other five rites consistently till he experiences the power of his virility. When he experiences the first "full bloom of youth" he can go ahead and learn the sixth rite."

In the sixth rite, the sex currents of the body are upturned – i.e. they are made to flow in an upward direction. The Colonel insists that the practitioner must be absolutely sure that he wishes to lead the life of a mystic. He must be absolutely sure in his mind and in his heart that this is what he desires in life, and then go ahead and learn the sixth Tibetan rite. The benefits of the sixth rite are bound to benefit him.

# The Essence Of The Sixth Rite

The colonel goes on to explain the essence of the sixth rite in detail in the booklet. He says that:

- The life energy/prana flows in the downward direction in average virile men.

- In order to gain super powers or mystic powers, these life forces need to be turned in the upward direction.

- Turning these powerful life forces in an upward direction is actually a very simple matter if done under expert guidance.

- Men over centuries have made futile attempts to master this procreative life energy force by either suppressing it or dissipating it.

- The key lies in transmuting it while simultaneously lifting it upward.

- When the sixth rite is practiced correctly, this life force is used effectively (not suppressed or dissipated) and the practitioner would have discovered the "elixir of life".

- This was something that even our learned well-versed ancestors were unable to do or experience.

- The sixth rite must be performed only when the student has an excess of procreative energy, which can be gained by practicing the first five Tibetans rites consistently.

- The sixth rite is very easy and can be performed at any time anywhere.

- It is imperative that the complete sequence of breathing exercises be repeated three times after doing the sixth rite.

### *How the sixth rite works:*

- We have more than 72,000 nadis in our body. The life energy/prana flows through these nadis.

- Kundalini is a reservoir of psychic energy that is found at the base of our spine. It is coiled up like a snake.

- When the Kundalini awakens, we experience a sense of pure joy, love and knowledge.

- Our consciousness expands as we become aware of the Divine Truth.

- We have three bandhas in our body: the mula bandha, the uddiyana bandha (6th rite) and the jalandhara bandha.

- These three bandhas function as energy valves for the life energy/ prana that flows within our body.

- When these three bandhas are activated by the Tibetan exercises, during meditation or while practicing other yoga postures or breathing practices the Maha bandha is formed.

- When these bandhas work together, the blocked life energy/prana is released and it starts flowing freely nourishing that particular area.

- These bandhas also bind the life energy/prana within the body to avoid dissipation.

- This life energy/prana gets redirected within our body, thereby healing and rejuvenating us.

- When this life energy/prana starts flowing freely and in the correct direction, it makes us aware of the neuro-physical and mental energy patterns of our physical body.

- The Uddiyana bandha (sixth rite) is a valve that opens upwards during the flow of life energy.

- While doing the sixth rite, the blocked energy starts flowing upwards.

- When this energy starts flowing upwards, the psychic energy that is stored in the Kundalini is released.

- It can now flow freely and a direct connection is established between the base chakra and the chakra located in the crown.

## A word of caution:

- The expert guidance of a highly competent spiritual teacher is recommended while practicing this sixth rite.

- This rite involves the nervous system and if done incorrectly or without expert supervision one may experience mental instability or psychic disturbances leading to mental stress and suffering.

The connection between tantra and the sixth rite:

There seems to be a strong connection between tantric practices and the sixth Tibetan rite. A person practicing tantra uses the life energy/prana that flows through his own body and through the universe to achieve purposeful goals. The goals differ from person to person. Some people crave for material success while others yearn for spiritual progress. Most tantric practitioners feel that it is absolutely necessary to know and learn about mystical experiences.

The tantric practitioner uses Yoga, mantra chanting, mudras (hand gestures) meditation, mind training techniques etc to enhance the flow of prana/life energy. These practices should be made available only to students seeking advanced knowledge and who already have sound knowledge of basic practices. These advanced tantric practices should be done under the expert guidance of a guru to understand their potential.

Without the guidance of an expert, these tantric practices are likely to be misused or misinterpreted, which may prove to have disastrous consequences affecting the mental equilibrium and health of a person.

In fact, most tantric practices are kept a secret, mainly because they should never be practiced without proper guidance. Most people cannot even comprehend the symbolic and psychological impact that these practices have on one's body, mind and health. It is easy to misunderstand and misinterpret these practices and dismiss the guidance of an expert as unnecessary.

# Modification Of The Five Tibetan Rites

- One must always keep in mind that the original book was published in 1939 and Colonel Bradford learned these rites from the Tibetan monks who lived in the Himalayas. The level of their physical fitness must have been extremely good in order to survive the harsh weather conditions there.

- They cultivated and cooked their own food, which was totally organic, and all their physical activity kept them in top form.

- They probably started practicing these Tibetan rites from a very young age.

- In comparison, we seem to have led a sedentary life style and are not as physically fit as our ancestors.

- So these rites have gradually been modified to suit individual needs.

- Colonel Bradford makes a mention of this in the booklet and says that a few people create their own little supports or aids to help them while practicing these movements, and it is perfectly fine to do so.

- He narrates an example of an old Indian man who just couldn't get the correct posture of the fourth rite even once. He would not be content with just lifting his body off the floor. He wanted it to parallel to the floor exactly like the rite prescribed. So he started working with a ten-inch tall box, which was about two and a half feet long. He padded it with bedding. He then lay down flat on his back on the bed with his feet and hands touching the floor at either end. Now he found it extremely easy to lift his body to the horizontal position. Colonel Bradford endorses modifying the exercises to suit the requirements of our body as long as the core of the exercises is not tampered with.

- As long as no radical changes are made that may have an adverse effect on the spin rate of the chakras, it is okay to modify them as per our bodily requirements.

- It is imperative that we remember one fact: The prime priority of any form of exercise, including the five Tibetan rites, should be safety and achievability.

- Several thousands of people practice the modified forms of Tibetan rites regularly.

- When broken down into a series of steps, they build up our strength gradually and safely.

- Right from day one, the prime focus should always be on correct alignment. This way, we learn to perform the exercises correctly and prevent the occurrence of muscular imbalances.

- A gradual build up of our core stability takes place. This activates the deepest muscles of the trunk while protecting and stabilizing the spine.

- The modified exercises prevent us from straining or injuring our lower back or neck.

- When we build up our strength gradually, we learn to do the movements using our strength and coordination instead of relying on the momentum of the movement.

- Additional energy breathing sessions enhances the effect and impact of the five Tibetan rites on our body.

# Tibetan Medicine

After knowing about the Tibetan Rites, it's time to learn about the ways by which Tibetan Medicine can cure diseases. The good thing about it mainly is the fact that your healing will be natural-- 100% safe, and 100% effective.

What is Tibetan Medicine?
Tibetan Medicine is perhaps one of the oldest traditional forms of healing. Experts say that Tibetan Medicine has been practiced for over 4 thousand years, mostly in Tibet and other Himalayan regions.

The real Tibetan language for this form of healing is "Sowa Rigpa". Sowa translates to "healing what is not in balance" and Rigpa meaning "The science or the knowledge".

Another important note that you should learn about is the knowledge of the 5 sciences in Tibetan culture. The following are the important sciences: Logic, Philosophy, Study of Sounds, Technology, and Medicine, which is the Sowa Rigpa.

Guess what? Among all these sciences, Sowa Rigpa is hailed as the most important one.

The Principle Behind The Tibetan Medicine
In healing according to the ways of Sowa Rigpa, there are three factors: the human body, the disease that damages it, and the treatment. The important thing to note is this: all these factors have one thing in common-- they are ruled by 5 elements. These elements are the following: earth, fire, water, space, and air.

These 5 elements are working alone and together in harmony to bring peace (or health) in the body. So, when one of the elements becomes disturbed or imbalanced (may be it has become deficient, or may be it becomes excessive), then not only will that single element be affected badly, but also the other elements.

Since the cause of the health issue is the disturbance in one (or more) of the elements, the cure will be to balance them out using diet. The diet, however, will not be generalized. In fact, the regime will be based on the person himself.

To give you an overview, here is a list of the healing methods employed in Tibetan Medicine:
- Use of herbs

- Blood donation

- Heat and/or cold application

- Tibetan Moxa

- Enema

- Medicinal bath

- Massage

In Depth Explanation of the 5 Elements

In this section, we will have an in depth knowledge about the 5 elements of the Sowa Rigpa. This piece of information is important in healing so it is best to memorize them by heart. Another alternative is to bookmark this page of the book in times when something is wrong with your health.

Air - Just the quality and the function of air already give you the heads up of what part it will be most connected to: the respiratory system. Should the air element be imbalanced, a person may have difficulty in breathing, and it will often be caused by lung problems.

Another important characteristic of air is this: it can be felt. So a deficiency or excess can mean you will have skin problems, or in a broader view, it can cause disturbance in the way you feel for things-- both physically and intangibly.

Fire - The fact the symbol of heat, it is connected with how the body regulates the temperature. Should there be disharmony with this element; a person may start having problems in her tissues and organs. Why? It's because warmth signifies the continuous flow of blood. Lack of it can therefore impede the circulation.

Another notable characteristic of fire is it gives off light. If the fire is gone, a person may experience eye problems. Pallor or lack of color can also be due to this element's disharmony.

Water - If fire signifies the circulation, water represents the fluid part of the body, or to be more specific, the blood. According to Tibetan medicine, water is also the element responsible for taste, and the development of the fetus during conception (remember that a baby in the womb is surrounded by the amniotic fluid).

Space - Space is often associated with sound, seeing than an empty space sometimes gives off an echo or vibration. Thus, a disharmony to this element can cause hearing problems.

It is also connected with the empty spaces of our pores. And to make it even more appealing, space can give you the freedom to move. A deficiency or excess of this element can give you problems with mobility.

Space is also associated with rooms, or particularly, rooms to improve, grow, and mature.

Earth - Just as the earth is the ground where we stand at, the body part it represents also functions the same way. In other words, earth is connected with out bones (the framework), and the flesh that gives us form.
And remember how some people often comments about liking how the fresh earth smells? Fun enough, earth is also the element associated with our sense of smell.

The Three Nyepas
If the 5 elements are considered to be good, so long as they are well and balanced, the Tibetan Medicine also posits that our body also has bad elements that can cause harm.
Much like the 5 elements, these Nyepas (rLung, Tripa, and Peken) also work in harmony, however, unlike the 5 elements, they are very sensitive and if one of them becomes

disturbed, the other two will also be put to imbalance. And this imbalance will manifest as different signs and symptoms of ailments.

Traditional doctors of the Sowa Rigpa relates that Nyepas as three close knit brothers. According to them, these brothers are so tightly bonded that when one is feeling unwell, or is attacked, the other two will lose their good thinking, cause a severe disharmony.

# The Flow of Tibetan Medicine

The next part of the Tibetan Medicine discussion will be all about the objectives of Sowa Rigpa, what can be its benefits for the wellbeing of a person, causes of diseases, diagnosis, and treatment methods.

The Goals of Tibetan Medicine
What make Tibetan medicine more promising are the goals that it has. Unlike other practices that just seek to cure once the disease has descended upon the person, Sowa Rigpas seeks to prevent diseases from ever happening. In other words, it aims to make the person as healthy as possible so that ailments will not come his or her way.

Other goals also consist of improving the life span of people, and ensuring that a person's goals to become fit (holistically) are achieved. Lastly, should a disease happen, the Tibetan Medicine goal is to cure it safely and naturally.

Now these may seem like generic goals but are in fact, what makes Tibetan medicines some of the most sought after in the world. It is the specific and targeted goals that make the medicines a good option for all those that are looking to prevent the occurrence of an illness and maintain good health and vigor.

What are the benefits of Tibetan Medicine?
The main benefit of Tibetan Medicine is its holistic approach in health. If a person becomes sick, the root of the disease will be treated, but the healing will not stop there. The goal, as we have mentioned, is to bring overall health, so other measures to make sure that the disease, or other diseases, will not come upon that person, will be taken.

More than that, Sowa Rigpa also aims to have the mentality and spirituality healthy. Due to this, Tibetan Medicine is a very effective approach for the following diseases or conditions:

1. Can be used to prepare a person for a chemotherapy or radiation session. Subsequently, it can be used during and also after the treatment. This is because chemo can take a toll on the body and it is important to prepare it to take it on.
2. Perfect for people who are trying to recover their strength and energy. Have you noticed how weak you can get at times, maybe it is because of a lack of vitality and vigor and so, it is best for you to try these medicines and fix this problem.
3. Joint pains. Especially if you have arthritis or rheumatoid arthritis, it is important for You to try these medicines and avail relief from your problems.
4. Problems in a person's digestive system like food poisoning. With the types of food that we put into our bodies these days, it is only normal that we feel like a lot of unnecessary junk is circulating inside out bodies. The

best way to treat this is by taking up Tibetan medicine and finding a feasible solution to the problem.

5. 5. If a person is having reproductive malfunctions (particularly for women), Sowa Rigpa can also be employed. Tibetan Medicine is good for problems in menstruation (such as irregularity and dysmenorrhea). So it is a viable option to consider it if you have a condition such as pcod. It is a much better option as compared to English medicine and you can avail better relief from it.

6. Also good for mothers and their babies because Tibetan Medicine also caters to prenatal and postnatal care. Many mothers feel weak after giving birth and will need to regain their strength. Similarly, young babies will need to develop their strength and turn healthy. All this can be remedied by taking up Tibetan medicines.

7. Sinus problems, more particularly congestion. This usually happens if a person has a deviated septum. There will be all sorts of problems such as nose block and wheezing. But the best solution to all this is to take up Tibetan medicine and find viable solutions to the problem.

8. Lung and other respiratory ailments from something as common as cough and cold, to something as big as bronchitis and pneumonia.

9. Neurological disorders: motor impairments, multiple sclerosis, sciatica, and nerve compression.

10. Heart illnesses.

11. Skin diseases.

12. Endocrine problems such as diabetes.

13. Liver problems such as hepatitis.

14. Psychological issues like depression, anxiety, and frustration.

15. Insomnia

16. Other chronic diseases.

# Causes of Diseases According to Tibetan Medicine

Tibetan Medicine also incorporates some of the teachings of Buddhism, thus, the causes of diseases can be narrowed down to the principle of cause and effect.

This cause and effect notion can be further broken down into two categories: The long-term causative factors and the short term ones.

Long-term causative factor suggests that a person may experience illnesses if he or she ignores being healthy, and is always subjected to the three Nyepas or poisons of negative feelings. These negative feelings are the following:

- Desires can cause a person to have the Nyepa rLung

- Hatred paves the way for Tripa, and

- Ignorance causes Peken

The short-term causative factors are those with immediate causes, such as injury and trauma, or improper eating habits.

# Diagnosis in Tibetan Medicine

When it comes to pointing out the disease or condition a person has, Tibetan Medicine resorts to three simple methods that you can do on your own, and at the comfort of your home.

Doctors of Sowa Rigpa analogize the diagnostic methods to a person predicting the weather. If the sky is blue and there are no clouds, the chances of raining are slim. If the sky is dark, and the clouds are looming, then rain will probably be in any minute.

These are the three diagnostic method used in Sowa Rigpa:
1. Observation
2. Touch or palpation
3. Questioning

Now, let us discuss them one by one:
Observation is a form of examination that uses all the 5 senses, but mostly the sense of sight. The funny part is, the

doctor also observes the patient's senses, and from there can come up with diagnoses.

Examples of diagnosis are the following:
1. Poor eyesight means that the patient is suffering from weak liver.

2. Should there be problems in his spleen, his lips can either be dry or sore.

3. Weak kidneys can manifest as hearing problems.

4. Problems with the heart can cause a person to have speech difficulties.

5. A patient with nasal problems can also have problems with his lungs.

More than that, other data are also collected such as weight and height and the person's complexion. Even the body language can give the person away if he is feeling stressed or pained.

Another branch observation in Tibetan Medicine is the examination of the tongue and urine.

First up, the tongue observation is related to the three Nyepas:
1. If the tongue is reddish in color, but has dry texture, and coarse to look at, the person is being violated with the Nyepa rLung.

2. If the tongue is coated with something thick and yellow, then the patient is having some problems with the Trispa.

3. If the tongue is pale in color, moist, and the coating it has is whitish, then the person is suffering from the Nyepa Peken.

Urine Examination
Wait up. If you feel that urine analysis is often done in the laboratory and you have to wait for minutes, or may be even hours, think again.

What's unique about Sowa Rigpa is that urine analysis is done on the spot, in front of the patient. What does a doctor look for during the urine exam? Well, to be honest, a lot of things such as bubbles, temperature, sediments, color, and smell.

The best time to inspect a patient's urine is upon waking, and under the natural light of the sun.

Touch or Palpation
Unlike the first one, it will need more training, may be even decades of studying and feeling. For Tibetan doctors, the pulse (the one being felt during the palpation) is a messenger from the disease itself toward the physician.

The best time to inspect the pulse is in the morning, when the patient just awakens, has not moved from bed yet, and has an empty stomach.

However, anytime of the day will also be accurate. The Tibetan Doctor may ask you to relax for a few minutes before taking your pulse.

The location of the pulse to be inspected also matters. Truthfully, the body has several pulse points. What's important is to locate the pulse point that is not too far, and not too close. Doing so will impede the message. For this reason, the doctors often inspect the radial artery because it is in the right position from all the major organs.

Questioning

Although it sounds so simple, the truth is the physician has to be very adept in questioning, never forgetting the important details. Among the three diagnostic method, questioning is the most informative and the one that has the power to build rapport.

# Components of Tibetan medicine

## *Acupuncture*

The Tibetan medicine was highly influenced by Indian medicines. This is because the Indians flourished in the field of medicine and this was propagated all through out the world. The Tibetans so happened to make use of all the medicines and procedures that the Indians followed and used it to their advantage. Right from homeopathy to Ayurveda, all branches of Indian medicine were exploited and the Tibetans picked up the best of each branch.

One such influence was that of acupuncture. In traditional Indian medicine, small sharp bamboo slivers were used to pierce through the skin and affect the pulse points present all over the body. These points would directly correspond to a particular part of the body and by stimulating these points;

the doctor could easily stimulate the organs. So if you were to experience pain in your joints, then the doctor would know where its pulse point lies and pierce it with a bamboo sliver. After some tome, the doctor would remove the pierced bamboo and the person's pain would slowly begin to deplete.

Similarly, small steel needles were introduced, which would be inserted into the skin. These needles would help stimulate the pulse points and reduce the pain in the particular organs. Although needles are widely used, many people still prefer to use the traditional bamboo sticks as they contain more power and help in dealing with the issue in the best possible manner.

The procedure starts out by cleansing the area where the pulse point is present and the needles are inserted with the help of plastic tubes that cover the top of the needle. The practitioner will know the exact time when the needle needs to be inserted and some experts check the pulse for exact time.

The insertion of the needle is supposed to be pain free but it will entirely depend on the level of expertise of the practitioner. If he is efficient enough, then the pain will be very less and if he is not efficient then there will a slight pain that will linger. The needles are about 3 centimeters in length and will pierce the skin to reach the pulse points and stimulate the various organs.

Acupressure is related to acupuncture and deals with stimulating the pulse points in a similar manner. But instead of invasive therapy, the doctor will either use a blunt instrument to press against the pulse points or do so with their bare fingers. Another branch of it is known as sujok therapy, which deals with affecting the various pulse points of the body using wooden and plastic pens and rollers that are rolled over the pulse points. Once you understand how these pulse points work you can start helping yourself at home and don't have to rely on an expert for help. The pulse points will mostly be present on your palm or under your feet. For example, the area behind your big toe is associated with your brain and by massaging this area; you will affect your brain's functioning.

Acupuncture is to only be performed by thorough professionals and not anybody else. It is vital that you check the credentials of the person before you decide to take up the treatment.

## *Chiropractic*

Apart from the Indian influence, there was also Chinese influence on Tibetan medicine. The Tibetan practitioners adopted various forms of Chinese medicines to formulate their medicines. One such practice is known as chiropractic, which is a part of Tibetan medicine. I am sure you have heard of this word before and wondered what it meant, well, here is an explanation of it.

Chiropractic is a form of alternate medicine, which is used to treat several ailments in the body, mainly in terms of body alignment and balance. The chiropractic uses techniques to affect the musculoskeletal framework of a person and aligns the spine. So he or she works by pressing the back in such a way that the spine is aligned and straightened. This straightening helps the person stand straight and also sit in a proper posture.

Many illnesses including that of the joints and other bones of the body is dealt with using chiropractic. So if you think you have problems in your back or bones, then visit chiropractor and you will notice a difference almost instantly.

The main philosophy behind chiropractic is that, the spine is the true indicator of a person's health. So if you have a healthy spine, then it means that you are healthy overall. So a chiropractor will first check your spine and its alignment and only then begin work on your body. Additionally, if he thinks some bones are out of place or not aligned, then he will set them for you.

Although there is no real pain involved, if the spine or any bones are stuck in a very stiff place, then it will hurt. So it is important to visit a professional chiropractic.

It is believed that these chiropractic practitioners have just as much power and authority as any medical doctor would and this is one alternate science that is considered to be extremely effective. However, you must not rely on this science alone and can use it as a supplementary practice along with these medicines.

In a standard chiropractic clinic, you will find a table where you have to sit on it or lie face down and the practitioner will press your back and spine to affect it. As soon as a "click" sound is heard, it means that the issue has been dealt with and everything is now in place. As soon as the spine is aligned, the person's health will start to improve and all the organs will work effectively.

It is believed that there are also some practitioners who work on animals and help them have their spine aligned. This is seen as a good treatment option for all those pets, who are allergic to medications. But you will have to find a professional animal chiropractic in particular and not a general one. Since those are rare, you must do a thorough background search for it before going through with it.

### Homeopathy

Homeopathy is a traditional form of Indian medicine, which is now an official part of Tibetan medicine. Homeopathy, in fact, is one of the widest practiced forms of traditional Tibetan medicine. It is something that is said to help in curing even the gravest of illnesses with much ease.

But it will take a lot more time than English medicine and so, should only be considered if the illness is not grave.

If you were to visit a professional homeopath, then he or she will give you a small cylindrical bottle containing small white or green pills. These pills are made from natural ingredients including green tea, herbs, roots, barks, flowers etc. All these ingredients contain powerful properties, which make them ideal to treat several human conditions.

Although there are some over the counter homeopathy medicines that are aimed at specific conditions, it is important to consult a professional homeopath, who will prescribe to you a specific medicine that will aim at your condition.

He practitioner will, in fact, mix two or three pills in a mortar and pestle and add the powder to a small bottle and give it to you. You must then add some to a glass of water and ingest.

It is important that you consult only a professional homeopath and check their certificate and make sure that they know what they are doing. Usually, these practitioners will not publicize their business and will be hard to find. So the best way to find a good one is by asking some one if they know of anyone who is good and whether they have availed any relief themselves.

Another similar form of practice is known as Ayurveda. This practice is a lot like homeopathy and deals with using natural ingredients to cure a condition. It prescribes similar tablets except that they will not be small and white. They can be of any color but will not be coated unlike English medicine. They will be raw and in their natural state.

Again, you must consult an Ayurveda expert who is a thorough professional and has been practicing since long. If he does not have a certificate of authenticity, then it is best that you not consider him at all.

They should also operate under a valid license and not simply pose as a practitioner. The time taken to see results might not be as quick as English medicine and might take some time. Many people prefer to use this treatment in addition to English medicines, which will help add leverage to their practice.

### Naturopathy

Naturopathy is a form of Tibetan medicine practice, which employs all natural forms of treatment including homeopathy and also herbalism. There are several naturopathy therapy centers all over the world and you will surely find one in and around your area. All you have to do is look for one online and avail treatment for your condition.

Right from internal to external issues and also weight loss problems, naturopathy has a solution for everyone. They will give you both internal medicine and also external stimulation to help solve your issue.

This external situation can include bathing in natural springs or immersing yourself in natural mud, smearing yourself with salt, bathing in the sun, meditating, crystal healing etc. All these are just a few of the things that are suggested as treatment options and there are many more.

There are many people who believe that naturopathy is the best way to lose weight without having to expressly exercise for it. All it takes is attending a course and availing the naturopathy treatments.

Many centers have all types of treatment facilities available and will be well equipped with all the things that are needed to treat someone. They are generally quite expensive, owing to their popularity and how there are many testimonials available claiming their effectiveness in treating the various illnesses.

But like any of the other treatment options, you will have to check for a valid license and see if they are authorized to carry out the various treatments. You can choose a place that has good reviews or something that has a lot of recommendations.

Although many people have questioned the effectiveness and use of the therapies prescribed as per naturopathy, there is no evidence to prove otherwise and so, many people continue to avail treatment. It is best that you do your own research before taking up any treatment and know exactly what you are getting yourself into.

Apart for these, there are also several other forms of Tibetan medicine including siddha, osteopathy and many such sciences. Each one is quite unique and known to help people with their issues.

You must take it up seriously if you want to avail relief from your conditions. If you have faith in the therapies then it will work better. This is because the mind and body are connected at a very deep level and you cannot fully understand how the two operate. It is not like these will not work for all those that don't believe in it but those who do will experience better results. So if you adopt these practices with an open mind, then you will realize that it makes a lot of sense and how one thing is always attached to another. All those who believe in the practice will definitely experience better results.

# Treatment in Tibetan Medicine

The common misconception that patients have is this: curing them is solely the job of the doctor. If the disease was not cured, then it is the doctor's fault. That sort of outlook is exactly the reason why most treatment methods (modern or traditional) fail.

Treatment in Tibetan Medicine also posits that healing is a team effort. Should the doctor advise you to change something in your lifestyle, and then you should try your best to abide by the changes prescribed. If he asks you to take medications, then you have to take the right medications, at the right time, and at the dose that he told you to. If you fail to follow these basic rules, then you will not make a lot of headway and wonder if the doctor was right in the first place. Similarly, if you don't follow the course mapped by Tibetan medicines, then you will not be able to see remarkable results.

## Modification in the Diet

Doctors practicing Tibetan Medicine believes in this: People are overfed, but are certainly under nourished. Why? It's because the process of food production took a turn not for the better, but for the worse.

Through the years, the freshness of the foods prepared in out table has diminished drastically. Each spoonful of meals is filled with chemical preservatives, artificial food colorings, unhealthy antibiotics, etc.

For this reason, Tibetan Medicine demands that a person resort to organic eating. Organic eating refers to eating fruits and vegetables that have been grown organically. If these fruits and vegetables have been grown in soils laden with chemicals, then it is obvious that they will be thoroughly unhealthy. And yet we end up eating them, as we will not have a choice.

## Medications in Tibetan Medicine

If there is something that makes Tibetan Medicine so unique, it is their way of prescribing and preparing medications. Physicians make use of different ingredients, not just herbs. A patient's medicine can comprise of soil, wood, metals, gems and crystals. Yes that is right, it is extremely unique and something that is only available in Tibetan medicine. It is not only about tablets and syrups and there is use of all the main elements and the right combination of these that is employed to help people.

Depending on the need, a patient's medicine can make use of just 2-3 ingredients, but if gravely needed, a single dose can have as many as 150 ingredients.

## The General Idea in Tibetan Medicine

Although prescription and preparation of medicine according to Tibetan practice takes time and expertise, you can have a general idea of what to take depending on the Nyepa that you are having problems with. Follow these simple guides:

1. If you are having problems with the Nyea rLung, you should prepare medications that combine the taste of sweetness, saltiness, and sourness.

2. Problems with Trispa can be remedied using medications that taste both bitter and sweet.

3. Imbalance in the Peken should be prescribed with medications that are both sour and salty.

## The Use of Elements in Treating the Nyepas

As for using the elements to treat the problems caused by Nyepa, follow these guides:

- The element earth, due to its grounding capacity, can remedy problems with rLung because this Nyepa is light and very movable. However, earth can worsen problems with Peken because the two share almost the same heavy qualities.

- Like earth, water can also aggravate Peken, but it can remedy problems with Trispa.

- Fire, on the other hand can worsen the problems with Trispa, but it can remedy your difficulties with Peken. This is because fire is warm and Peken is cool in nature.

- Air can pacify any discord with Peken, but it can aggravate rLung.

## 7 *Procedures in Tibetan Medicine Preparation*

1. Plants to be used as ingredients in medications should be well taken cared of. For example, if its natural habitat is cold climate, it should have grown there and likewise if its habitat is a warm environment. The soil should be healthy and there should not be any harmful fertilizer.

2. Collection should be made appropriately. In Tibetan practice, for a plant to be an effective ingredient, it should be harvested at the right time. But to make things more complicated, different parts of the plants have different times of harvesting, and those times should be followed as well.

3. Detoxification must be performed. Like men, plants should also be detoxified. And to do that, the toxic parts should be removed after harvesting. Although the toxic part will not be fatal to the patient, it can cause digestive upset.

4. Plants should be sorted and dried. As simple as it sounds, this step is in fact very complicated. This includes choosing which plants to be collected, and the doctors must have the knowledge about the plant's characteristics.

5. There is a timeframe. While some of them effectiveness will remain, older plants will be less potent to cure illnesses, so Tibetan Medicine often discard medications that have plant ingredients not harvested on the same year.

6. Another complicated step is to follow a certain formula in preparing the medications. This is done so that the medications will be easier to digest.

7. Compounding the medication.

### How do you take Tibetan Medicine?

The end product of the medicine is usually in pill form. But unlike other pills, there is a preparation before you can take it. First, depending on the prescription, you must place 1 or 3 pills in a cup and fill the cup with water. Soak the pills for 30 minutes before taking it.

For busy people however, doctors suggest that you soak the pills overnight. Take it in the morning (crush it in your mouth) after brushing your teeth.

As for the storage, the pills already come in bottles with tight caps. Make sure that you tightly cover the bottles so as not to expose them to air; doing so will preserve the potency of the drugs.

It may not taste that good but just think about how natural your medications are! They do not contain any form of preservative!

# The Tibetan Massage

Just like other treatment program, Tibetan Medicine also offers its own brand of therapeutic massage. Tibetan Massage is termed as Ku Nye (pronounced as Coo-nye), and has been practiced in Tibet and other parts of the Himalayan region for over a thousand years.

### What can you expect on a Tibetan Massage?

The name Ku Nye stands for 2 words that underline what is to be expected of the massage. Ku means oil, and Nye means giving pressure. Thus, Tibetan massage will use oils to put pressure to a certain spot in the body that is responsible for the illness the patient is feeling.

However, unlike other massage, the oils used in Ku Nye are natural. It can be from butter, olive oil, sesame oil, olive oil, sandalwood oil, and the like.

Also, after the massage is over, the healer shall perform a cleansing activity called ChiPa. ChiPa is done by placing different types of powder on the body parts so that the oil used will be absorbed.

## *What are the benefits of Tibetan Massage?*

Ku Nye is beneficial for people who are suffering from the following:

1. Foot pain
2. Skin problems, primarily if your skin is dry and rough in texture
3. Circulatory system problems, or if the condition you have is caused by poor circulation
4. Whiplash and rigidity in the muscles of the body
5. Constipation
6. Backaches
7. Health problems that may have risen due to stress level

It is also important to understand that Ku Nye can be a reliable stand-alone treatment, but there will be a better effect if you follow it up with the treatment the doctor may prescribe for you.

## *Contraindications to Ku Nye*

While Tibetan Massage is very effective, it still has several contraindications. Please avoid from undergoing the Ku Nye if you are troubled with the following:

1. Inflammatory diseases or any disease that are caused by infection
2. Water retention
3. Diseases that originate from the liver or gallbladder

# Tibetan Medicine and Physical Decay

What makes Tibetan Medicine both scientific and mystifying is the ability of the physician to determine physical decay using several signs. The scary part is that physical decay often means death.

Basically, there are 4 signs, and we will discuss them one by one.

### 1. Long Term Signs

Long-term signs of decay can be observed through one's dreams, actions, thoughts, and even physical appearance. Let's talk about the dreams first.

### Dreams

Dreams, according to Tibetan Medicine can be classified into several types, depending on what is happening within the dream.

For example, if you have seen something during the day and it manifests itself in your dream-- that is called a seeing dream. It goes if you have heard, or touched something. There can also be praying dreams, which is dreaming of something you constantly desire to have.

In this book, however, we will only discuss 2 types of dreams: the positive and the negative ones. This is because these two are connected in the manifestation of physical decay, death, or health.

## List of negative dreams:

1.  Riding an animal, or worse, a corpse, while you are naked and your direction is southward
2. If you see your head growing out a tree, or if there is a bird's nest on your head, that's also a negative dream
3. Having a thorny plant grow from your heart, or when there is a lotus flower growing from your chest
4. Your skin is falling off
5. Shaving or cutting your hair while you ae naked
6. Sleeping in a cemetery
7. Being washed away by flood or being buried in the mud

Tibetan doctors say that if these dreams happen at the time of dawn, then they can be considered as signs of physical decay.

## List of positive dreams:
1. Wearing something clean, and white
2. Watching as the fire burns brightly
3. Meeting a master of some sort

4. Mountain climbing or when you are climbing a tree
5. Watching the blue ocean
6. Praised by parents
7. Swimming

Like the negative dreams, if they constantly happen at the time of the dawn, then these dreams signify good health, and may be even gains in the material arena.

## Thoughts and Actions

Switching from one personality to another is very indicative of physical decay. For example, a person who is normally easy to get along with becomes hateful, and hard, that person is most likely suffering from a grave illness. The same thing also applies if a person is normally very serious and then suddenly became happy.

Other doctors also suggest that a sudden change from behavior towards the doctor is a good sig of physical decay.

## Physical appearance

Physical signs of decay are not delivered from the diagnosis section; in fact they are more like manifestations. Examples of physical signs of decay are the following:

1. Seeing yourself headless in front of the mirror, or when you see yourself missing a limb
2. Seeing that your shadow suddenly disappears even when the sun is shining directly above you
3. When taking a bath, you have noticed that your whole body is wet, but the area in your chest where your heart should be is dry

4. Not hearing the sounds of your knuckles when you crack them, but before there were audible sounds

## *2. Short Term Signs*

Short-term signs are examined through a person's senses. Should there be a reduction in the effectiveness of the senses, then it can be considered as short-term physical decay.

Example is when the vision suddenly blurs, or when the hearing stopped being effective.

## *3. Uncertain Signs*

Uncertain signs happen when negative dreams take place during the time of severe illness, but they also disappear after the illness is cured.

The reason why it is uncertain is because signs are usually persuasive. They do not disappear, but in this case, they did-- right after the ailment also disappeared.

## *4. Certain Signs*

Certain signs are signs that an individual shows physically, like not being able to take in food, being nothing but muscles and bones, and having no positive response to the most potent of treatment.

Certain signs are also definitive; you can see them the moment that death is looming. Just imagine a person having no pulse--that is a certain sign of decay or death.

# How to Deal With Diseases

When a person contracts an ailment, the physician cannot diagnose right away, and thus cannot delve into a much potent treatment plan unless the cause of the problem is pinpointed as the root.

- The truth is, after an initial observation, the physician might prescribe a certain medication first, based of course, on what he feels is the disease.

  For example, the patient shows signs of having imbalanced Trispa, so the doctor will give her the medication for it. If the patient responds well to the initial treatment, then the doctor will know for sure that the cause of the disease is that Nyepa.

- From then on, he con now describe FULLY what the disease is, its signs and symptoms, what is to be expected during treatment, and of course, the treatment itself.

- Should the patient have a deep fever that is interfering with the treatment, the physician should find a way to release the heat from that hidden fever before proceeding to the actual treatment.

- Continuity is important. In cases where the patient already consulted another doctor, but the treatment fails, the current doctor should be given all the information about the previous treatment. He or she will have to determine where the treatment went wrong.

- The 4-Water therapy is performed in cases of severe illnesses that need immediate treatment. Four water therapy is a procedure where in the patient is instructed to 1) fast with food and only taking in water, 2) cooling the temperature down by having cold water baths, 3) taking in medications that are in liquid form, such as camphor concoction, and 4) performing a blood letting surgery, most commonly at the jugular brain.

- In cases of minor ailments, 4-water therapy is not necessary. In fact, the doctor may not suggest any medication, only resorting to modifying the diet, habits, behavior, and attitude.

- Individuality of Nyepas. The doctor will make it a point to isolate the problems of the Nyepas IF the problem is truly singular. For example, if the problem is only with the Trispa, the doctor will find curing ways so as not to bother the rLung and Peken.

- If the problems, however, are a combination from the three Nyepas, the physician must always initiate "peace between the Nyepas" in his treatment. Thus, the treatment is not isolated, but connected.

The patient is a very important factor. Last but not the least, Sowa Rigpa has it that the patient should be the core of the treatment. Everything will depend on the patient's constitution and structure.

# Chakras Explained

The Tibetan rites will help maintain the spin rate of the chakras no doubt, but it is important to cleanse the chakra from time to time to ensure that there are no blockages in it. These blockages can occur due to many external factors including injury or fall and internal injuries due to changes in emotions and the influence of stress. In this chapter, we look at what blockages in these chakras can do and why it is important to cleanse the chakras from time to time.

The blockages can be checked by making use of a clear quartz crystal. You must attach the crystal to a normal chain and hold it over the chakras. If it is turning properly, then it means the chakras are functioning properly. But if the crystal does not turn or turns anti clock wise, then it means the chakra is blocked. Once you know which chakra is blocked, you can start cleansing it.

## First chakra

The first chakra in the body is located behind the pubic bone and in front of the anus. This chakra deals with people being grounded. It also signifies strength and having the courage and confidence to move forward in life. The first chakra is said to help balance the rest of the chakras in the body. It is important for you to balance this chakra and cleanse it from time to time. The best way to cleanse this chakra is by consuming root vegetables. You can also lie down on the floor and remain as connected to the round as possible. There is also the stone cleansing that can be taken up. This refers to placing a colored stone above the area of the chakra and covering it with a small wooden or cardboard pyramid to trap the energy inside it. You can make this pyramid yourself or buy one. The stone associated with this chakra is hematite, which is a black stone.

## Second chakra

The second chakra is located at about a centimeter below the navel. This chakra helps in keeping your sexuality and sexual desires in check. If this chakra is operating properly then you will have confidence and be an extrovert. But if this chakra is not operating properly then you will feel like an introvert and not have the confidence to meet people. It is important to fix this chakra as it can also have an impact on your reproductive organs. The best way to fix this chakra is by exploiting your sexual desires and sorting out your emotional problems. If you keep feeling emotional and giving into them then you will suffer from all types of problems. The stone associated with this chakra is carnelian, which is a reddish stone. You can place it above the chakra and cover it with a pyramid. Allow it to stay there for at least 20 minutes.

### *Third chakra*

The third chakra is located below the sternum. This chakra is all about confidence, power and leadership. You need to cleanse this chakra if you want to enhance your leadership qualities. The third chakra also deals with you attaining your life's ambitions. Those that have a blocked chakra will not be able to exploit their ambitions and not have the capacity to display their true power. A blockage can also signify stomach problems and so it is important to cleanse it from time to time. The stone associated with this chakra is citrine. Place the citrine stone over the chakra and place the pyramid on top. You can also wear a chain with a citrine pendent such that it reaches the solar plexus chakra. This will ensure that the chakra is always turning properly.

### *Fourth chakra*

The fourth chakra is located next to the heart. This chakra is all about love and emotions. It helps you connect to other human beings and also to your lover. A blocked chakra will indicate your inability to connect with others and the need to find your true emotions. It is important to cleanse this chakra if you want to avoid any relationship issues that you are having with your spouse. The fourth chakra also deals with socializing and having a good connection with the various people in your life. The stone associated with this chakra is rose quartz, which is a beautiful pink stone. Place it over the chakra and cover it with a pyramid. Allow it to cleanse the chakra and if you don't have the time for this, then you can wear a chain and help place the stone right over the chakra. You will find that all your emotional and relationship problems have disappeared.

## *Fifth chakra*

The fifth chakra is located in the throat and deals with your communication capacity and how well you communicate with others. A blocked chakra can mean having both speech and hearing problems and an inability to communicate with others. So it is important to have this chakra fixed and remove all the blockages from it. The fifth chakra is to be cleansed regularly as it is associated with the thyroid gland. The stone associated with this chakra is the sodalite. The sodalite should be placed over the throat and covered with the pyramid. Allow it to stay there for at least 30 minutes. You can also place a short chain around your neck with the stone. Once the chakra is cleansed, you will find that your health is improving over all.

## *Sixth chakra*

The sixth chakra is located between your eyebrows. It is also known as the third eye chakra. This chakra deals with intellect and the ability to think properly. It also deals with foresight and decision-making. If there is a blockage here then the person will suffer from a lack of intelligence or the capacity to make good decisions. The best way to cleanse this chakra is by placing an amethyst in between the eyebrows and covering it with the pyramid. This will ensure that the energy is trapped inside the area. You will find that it is easier for you to make all the decisions in your life. You will also find yourself being much more intellectual and having the capacity to make good decisions in your life.

### Seventh chakra

The last chakra is place just above your head and is known as the aura chakra. The aura chakra deals with spirituality and your capacity to connect with the divine. You have to cleanse it from time to time to cleanse your aura. We will look at the aura in detail in the next chapter. The stone associated with this chakra is the clear quartz. You must place the clear quartz over your head and cover with the pyramid in order to cleanse this chakra. You will feel that your life is bettering and you are in a position to look towards your spiritual side and exploit it.

These form the various chakras in your body, which as you know are electromagnetic wheels that spin at a regular speed.

# Human Aura

The human aura is an electro magnetic field that is present around all human beings. This aura is a result of the chakras and the way that they spin. The aura is extremely strong when the person is completely healthy and is quite weak when the chakras are not spinning properly. So apart from getting the different chakras fixed, it is also important to get the aura to remain intact and in perfect condition.

The best way to get your aura checked is by getting a photograph taken of your electromagnetic rays. It is possible for you to see your aura with your naked eye. All you have to do is sit in sunlight and observe your hand and then your feet. Once you successfully see the aura in these parts, you can stand in front of a mirror and see your entire body's aura. You can also get someone else to look at it. A psychic will be able to see it easily and give you a diagnosis as soon as possible.

Once you know which part of the aura is affected, you can work towards cleansing the chakra that is causing that particular light in your aura to fade. These colors are red for the base chakra, orange for the second chakra, yellow for the third chakra, green for the fourth chakra, light blue for the fifth chakra, indigo for the sixth chakra and purple for the last chakra. Sometimes, these colors will not be brightly colored and they will fade over time. But for a normal young person, they will be bright enough.

Your aura will define how healthy you are and there will be different colors and patterns. If there is a dominant color like light violet, then it means that the person is having an awakening or enlightenment and the top most chakra is causing it.

There are many ways in which you can cleanse your aura and this is just as important as cleansing your chakras. Like Hindu philosophy, the Tibetans also believe that the aura of a person needs to remain clean and healthy and here are some ways that are prescribed to cleanse your aura.

The best way to cleanse and expand it is by spending some time under the sun. This refers to playing under the bright sun and cleansing your body thoroughly. All your chakras will start to rotate properly and you will feel completely rejuvenated.

The next best way to cleanse your chakra is by dropping

some sea salt from above your head and allowing it to trickle down the body. You must use good quality sea salt alone and nothing else. But be careful as some of the crystals can be sharp and hurt your head or body.

You can have a cold shower when you wish to cleanse your aura after a day out. If you think you have spent some time outdoors with other people, who probably rubbed off some of their negative energy on to you. You can also decide to take a dip in your tub by filling it with cold water. But don't do this if it is cold outside or you have a cold.

You can also rub some pure earth on your body to get rid of negativity. This pure earth is available in the form of fullers earth or you can also collect some red or black soil and add in some water to make a paste and then apply it all over your body. You can follow it up with a cold shower.

It is also a good idea to burn some sage leaves and then hold the bowl close to your body. The smoke is supposed to cleanse your aura and fix any of the problems present in it. You can also burn some thyme or any such herb that is readily available to you.

Another good method is by applying essential oil to your body. These essential oils are natural oils that are pressed from natural ingredients and you can easily stain your skin with these. The pleasant fragrance will keep lingering and help you feel good about yourself.

These form the various ways in which you can cleanse your aura but there are more. You must preferably use only any one of these types and not do all of them at once. Once you know something is working for you, you must stick with it instead of moving to some other form of cleansing.

# FAQs On The Topic

The topic of Tibetan rites is quite unique and not something that many people are aware about. So it is obvious that many questions will pop into mind when they are trying to adopt the ritual. In this chapter, I will ask and answer a few of the common questions that get asked on the topic and these will surely help you understand the topic better.

### What are the Tibetan rites?

The Tibetan rites are a set of 5 exercises that the monks of Tibet have been practicing for thousands of years. The rites are a set of 5 specific exercises that aim at helping the body through its wear and tear and rejuvenate it from the inside out. The rites aim at the 7 chakras that are present inside your body and help them spin at a regular pace. These chakras often get blocked owing to external forces and so, it is important for you to cleanse them regularly. This you can do, by performing these rituals from time to time.

### *Is there any scientific backing for these?*

These rituals have been carried out for thousands of years and many scientists have studied it for at least half that time. When Colonel Bradford started propagating it and once it fell on the ears of scientists, they decided to conduct a research on the topic. They understood that these rites have the capacity to affect people's bodies and minds and have a positive impact on their living. They also saw how these monks remained young for longer and their bodies did not contain much fat. So scientifically speaking, it is possible for you to avail all these benefits and improve your mind, body and soul.

## What are its uses?

As mentioned earlier, it is possible for you to fix your mental and physical ailments by practicing these rituals. Just by performing these rites, it is possible for you to improve your chakra spin rate and fix any of the problems that are present in your body. Looking young is always an agenda topper for most women, and men alike. So just by adopting these rites, it is possible for you to look younger for longer. Colonel Bradford is said to have taken up thee rites because he was told that the Egyptians had found a "Fountain of youth" and that is what prompted him to exploit the 5 rites.

### *Is it really effective?*

Yes. It is extremely effective. The rites have shown remarkable differences in people's health once they took it up. You too can find a difference in your health by taking up the rituals and allowing your body a chance to not just have your physical ailments fixed but also cause your mental blockages to be eliminated. Each of the rites is aimed at a specific chakra in your body and helps in spinning the chakras properly. Don't keep thinking about the effects and simply carry out the rites to experience a new high in your life.

## Is it for anyone?

Yes. It is for anyone interested in losing weight and looking younger for longer. All you have to do is take up the rites and perform them regularly. There is no age or sex bar and anyone can perform it. Generally, it is observed that the endocrine system takes a toll at the time of puberty and so, youngsters can take it up to stabilize their body. It is also severely affected when a woman hits menopause and so, it is ideal for these women to take up the rituals in order to help the various chakras in their bodies rotate properly and avail relief from the various side effects of the endocrine changes.

## Can women of any age perform?

Women between 18 years and 45 years can perform it with ease. But those above that age need to consult a doctor and make sure that they can take up these exercises. The same extends to men and those above the age of 50 must check with their doctors to know if performing these rituals is a safe bet for them. Once the doctor gives the nod, the person can take up the rites and perform them on a regular basis. But everything needs to be done in moderation and over doing it is never advisable. Perform the rites in the prescribed manner and not over do it.

### How fast are results shown?

The results will come about gradually and accumulate. So if you are to perform the rites regularly in this month, then its effects will show in the next month and so on. So it is like laying the foundation to experience results in the coming future. You must take it up seriously and not casually. If you take it casually then it might not have a big impact on your body. Your body must readily accept the rites and there should come a time when you can easily perform them without putting in too much effort.

### Are there any precautions to observe?

Yes. As is for most things in life, it is important to observe precautions. These precautions are in terms of performing the rites in the correct manner, performing them at all the right times, performing them under supervision if you are a minor or a senior etc. Once you adhere to all these specifications, you will have the chance to make the most of your 5 rites and allow them to affect your body, mind and soul.

### Where is the best place to perform these rites?

These rites can be performed anywhere you like and that includes your house, park, office and even college. As long as you have a little privacy and enough space to get into the various positions, it is possible for you to perform them anywhere that you like. But it is best to perform in an open area as opposed to a concealed one and there should be fresh air blowing in.

# Mindfulness And The 5 Rites

The five rites as we know are exercises that are meant to keep the body healthy. But we need something that can supplement it to help avail mental health and that something is mindfulness.

Mindfulness is an activity, which helps people live longer. This is because, the person is able to concentrate on only one aspect of life at any given moment, which helps them maintain a steady focus. The mindfulness technique has been practiced for several centuries and has only been perfected. What we have today is a set of mindfulness excises that can be performed on a daily basis and will not require you to put in too much effort. The monks find mindfulness in every little activity that they perform on a daily basis and you'll be required to do the same.

### Mindfulness breathing

The very first thing to do is to breathe mindfully. Breathing mindfully refers to breathing in such a way that your attention is completely focused on your breath. Most of us breathe extremely shallow and end up wondering why we suffer from stress. So to effectively solve this issue, all you have to do is breathe from your stomach as opposite to the top of your lungs. Every time you inhale, visualize your stomach expanding like a balloon and when you exhale, your stomach should deflate. Keep this up and make sure you concentrate on your breath every time you breathe in and out.

## *Mindfulness showering*

Mindfulness showering is a technique where you have to concentrate on your showering. This means that you take time out to concentrate on your showering technique and also pay attention to all the small details. Start by switching on the shower and standing under it until all your hair and body is wet. Now pick up your soap bar and hold it close to your nose. Take in a long sniff and smell all the ingredients present in the soap. Allow your senses to experience a new high. Now rub the bar of soap all across your hand and observe the trail it leaves behind. Work up a lather and then do the same all through your body. Finish your shower and spend five minutes reflecting on it.

## *Mindfulness walking*

Mindfulness walking is a great way to relax your mind and body. To perform this excise, start by choosing a straight path to walk on. This can be the park or just your street. Ideally, you must do this early morning where the air is crisp and there is no one to disturb you. Start walking in a straight line and concentrate on your foot movement. Don't be distracted by the sounds of nature and simply focus on your body movement. Keep walking until you feel tired. Now sit on a bench and focus only on the sounds made by the birds. Cut every other form of noise out and maintain your focus only on the birds. Now start walking back home and concentrate only on your steps again.

## *Mindfulness cleaning*

Mindfulness cleaning refers to cleaning the house or cleaning the cupboard or kitchen and you need to pay key attention to it. Generally, when we perform these types of activities, we end up thinking about everything else in the world. But it is important to be absorbed in the moment and not have your mind wander here and there. If you are cleaning the carpet, then pay close attention to just that and nothing else. Similarly, if you are ironing clothes then pay attention only to that and nothing else. If you get distracted then immediately bring your focus back to your activity and have a physical sign like the snapping of fingers to help your attention return.

## *Mindfulness cooking*

Mindfulness cooking refers to cooking with your mind and not simply assembling a few things present in your kitchen. After we start cooking the same meal every day, we end up falling into a habit. But this habit needs to be broken and we need to pay keen attention to what we are cooking. As we know, as per the Tibetan rites, it is important for us to cook fresh meals with organic vegetables and concentrate on just one food category. So if you are cooking proteins today, then pay keen attention to it and make sure that you are cooking with your mind and heart. Don't have any distraction on like the television of the radio and concentrate in just the meal.

## Mindfulness exercise

Mindfulness exercise refers to exercising by concentrating only on your exercise routine. When we exercise, we end up concentrating on the music that is playing. But while doing so, the body will not be able to perform the exercises properly. So even if you have the music on, you must concentrate on your exercising and make sure that your mind is fully focused on it. When you do so, not only will your mind have the chance to remain fresh and focused, but it will also add leverage to your exercise, as your mind will force the various muscles in your body to burn the fat faster.

## Mindfulness counting

Mindfulness counting is a technique that is employed to remain focused in a bad situation and not allow the pressures to get to you. So the important thing is to start by having a set pattern like counting up or counting down. If you are counting up, then you can choose something like 1 to 60 or 1 to 100 and vice versa for counting down. It is important that you do not get distracted by anything, when you are counting and close your eyes when you are performing the activities. This is extremely useful if you have a stressful work on hand or have a big meeting coming up and need to relax your mind.

## Mindfulness dreaming

Mindfulness dreaming is a technique where you pay close

attention to your dreams. This means that you remain conscious when you are asleep or at least try to remember your dreams consciously when you wake up. Have a notebook and pencil handy with you and write down your dream. Your dreams are an indication of what lies inside your subconscious, as humans, it is important to unite the conscious and the subconscious and so, it is vital that you pay attention to your dreams. Once you have it written down for a month, read through all the dreams and try to establish a pattern. If you spot a problem thee then work towards solving it but if you see that your dreams are happy, then put in efforts to maintain the same type of lifestyle.

### *Mindfulness listening*

Mindfulness listening refers to listening to music or a song by paying key attention to it. Music and songs are great for both your body and mind. To perform this activity, start by picking a nice song or a tune. Now pay keen attention to it. Listen to all the small notes and each and every detail of it. Don't listen to some heavy music like rock or metal, as your mind will not. Be able to concentrate on it.

# The Importance Of Meditation And Its Types

Meditation is an important part of life. When a person meditates, he or she enables the mind, body and soul to unite. The Tibetan monks perform meditation on a daily basis and use it as a tool to maintain both mental and physical health. In this chapter, we will look at the different types of meditational practices that you can adopt and increase your overall well being.

## *Yoga mediation*

When it comes to yoga and meditation, the two go hand in hand. Although both are said to have originated in India, there is a subtle difference between the two. The difference being meditation is mental in nature and yoga being physical in nature. But there are a few breathing exercises that make use of both these concepts and they are explained as under.

### *Pranayama*

Pranayama is a breathing practice that helps in reducing stress and also aids in the intake of fresh oxygen. Just by performing pranayama, you can effectively reduce the amount of cortisol present in your brain. To perform this form of meditation, start by sitting with a straight back, legs folded and eyes closed. Now hold your right nostril tightly closed using your thumb. Breathe in through your left nostril and hold your breath. Now close your left nostril using your index finger and open up your right nostril. Now exhale the breath and wait for a couple of seconds before inhaling through your right again. Now hold the breath before exhaling through your left and closing the right. Continue doing so for 5 minutes and then relax.

### Kapalbhati

Kapalbhati is the other form of exercise that is prescribed as per yoga. For this, you must sit in the same position as before but take short and deep breaths that arise from your stomach. So you must focus on the exhale more than the inhale. Your stomach must move in and out in quick succession. Do this for 5 minutes and then relax your body. If at any time you feel like your breath is not completing then stop immediately. This exercise is not advised for those suffering from hypertension.

### *Transcendental meditation*

This is probably the most common type of meditation that is performed in this world. Transcendental meditation is said to have originated in India where the spiritual gurus would perform it to avail relief from their mental and physical ailments. This meditation then spread to Tibet, where the monks started adopting it and made it a part of their life. They would perform it on a daily basis and help their minds remain calm and peaceful. To perform this form of meditation, all you have to do is find a quiet corner for yourself and assume the lotus pose. This is a pose where you sit with a straight back and fold your legs. Place the backs of your palms on your knees and close your eyes. Now chant a mantra like Om or Hum and make sure you allow the vibrations of the words to pass through your entire body. Make sure your mind is focused on your breath and also your words. Do this for around 15 minutes a day and can do it twice a day.

### *Kundalini meditation*

Kundalini meditation is a great form of meditation, which is prescribed to cleanse your chakras. Just by performing this form of meditation, you can easily open up all your chakras and allow them to rotate at the ideal speed. Start by sitting in the lotus pose and close your eyes. Now imagine a small ball of light originating in your base chakra. This light is collecting all the negative vibes from it and then moving to the second chakra located below your navel. It then moves to the third then the fourth then the fifth, the sixth and finally to the seventh and then exits your body through your head. It effectively collects all the negatives vibes, as it grows in size, and allows only positive ones to remain back. Do this for around 15 minutes.

### Qi gong

Qi gong is a modified form of the kundalini meditation and involves pretty much the same principles. The only difference being that only three chakras are involved being the first, the fourth and the seventh. Imagine a ball of fresh air originating from your first chakra and then moving up to your fourth. It then moves to your seventh and back to your fourth or heart chakra and then to the basal or first chakra. This ball of air is extremely purifying and its primary function is to cleanse your chakras completely. Although only three are involved, it effectively cleanses all your chakras thoroughly and helps in removing all forms of blockages.

### Hypnosis

Hypnosis is a type of meditation where a person is sent into a trance and the subconscious is tapped into. As was mentioned earlier, both the conscious and the subconscious mind are extremely important for a person and uniting the two is the key to healthy living. A qualified hypnosis helps you travel into a trance and allows you to see what lies there. If you don't want to visit a hypnotist then you can self induce a trance by lying back and trying to go into a deep thought. But don't fall asleep as that will not account for your trance. Once you have induced a trance, see what lies in your subconscious and write it down. This is a lot like paying attention to your dreams.

### Guided visualization

Guided visualization is a technique that is used to recover from an ailment in the fastest time possible. For this, you must imagine yourself as sleeping in a fresh field with green grass and crisp air or seeing a bright light at the end of the tunnel or something that will help you get over your current state at a faster pace. Now say for example you are having stress. You will close your eyes and imagine yourself sleeping in a green field and relaxing yourself. All your stress and tension has left you and you are absolutely fine. This form of meditation will help you get over any ailment.

### *Walking meditation*

Walking meditation is a form of meditation where you can walk and meditate at the same time. So for this, choose a long path that is free from any obstructions. A park will work fine. Now every time that you put your left leg forward you must inhale and when you put your right leg forward then you must exhale. Concentrate on your breath. Keep doing this until you feel tired. The Tibetans make use of a clock that sounds an alarm every time that a foot needs to go forward and you can make use of a similar signal.

### *Mindfulness meditation*

Mindfulness is a type of meditational practice that has given rise to the mindfulness techniques. In this form of meditation, the focus can be an innate object but the idea is to maintain steady focus on it. So start by sitting in a quiet place and placing a plant or a similar object in front of you. Now close your eyes by 3/4ths and focus only on the object. Don't get distracted by anything else that surrounds you. Remain that way for at least 20 minutes and try not to blink. Break into a gentle smile along the way and allow the smile to remain for the rest of the session.

### *Heart beat meditation*

Heartbeat meditation is a form of meditation that is extremely soothing and relaxes your mind and body. To perform this type of meditation, all you have to do is sit in a comfortable position and close your eyes. Now place your right hand over your heart and imagine the heartbeat travelling from your palm to your body. It moves through all the organs and supplies fresh oxygen. All the cells in your body are rejuvenating and it is causing your body to feel fully relaxed.

### *Zazen meditation*

Zazen is a form of movement-based meditation much like walking meditation. In this form, you must sit with your legs folded under your body such that you butt places on the back of your feet. Now start rocking yourself forward and backward like a pendulum and maintain a constant motion. You must set a motion that is not too fast and not too slow. You can focus on your breath if you like but the idea is to make the motion the primary focus of the exercise.

These form the various types of meditational practices that you can adopt and better your living like the Tibetan monks.

# Yoga Poses That Complement The 5 Tibetan Rites

Yoga is a form of exercise that is performed to help the body relax, and the internal organs feel massaged. The art is said to have originated in India and then rapidly traveled the world over. The Tibetans adopted the practice and made it an important part of their life. In this chapter, we look at some of the best poses that you can perform to supplement and compliment the Tibetan 5 rites.

## Bridge pose

The bridge pose is one, which is great for your lower abdomen as well as your chest and back. This pose is great for all those looking to avail relief from a stiff back. The pose is easy to perform and will not take a lot of time to understand and master. To perform this pose, start by lying on your back and folding your legs. Now, with the help of your feet and shoulders lift up your mid section. Place your hands under the gap that your body creates and interlock the fingers. Stay in the upright position for a few minutes before lowering your body back down. Perform this exercise for around 5 minutes.

### *Bow pose*

The wheel pose is better known as the dhanurasan. To perform this pose, start by sleeping face down on the ground. Now draw in a deep breath and lift your legs in the air, backwards. With the help of your hands, push your upper torso upwards and backwards. Now catch hold of your feet using your palms and create a bow shape with your body. Remain in the bow position for a few seconds before letting go and relaxing again. If you have pain in your lower back then avoid this pose or go about it slowly. You can perform this pose for around 5 minutes daily.

### *Forward bend*

The forward bend is a very basic type of yoga pose but one that is known to be extremely beneficial. This pose is great for the entire body and particularly your stomach and reproductive organs. It also helps in stretching and strengthening the spine. To perform this pose, start by sitting on the floor with your legs stretched out and maintain a straight back. Now bend forward and try to touch your toes without bending your knees. You must feel a tight stretch in your hamstrings, which will help in strengthening them. As you progress with this exercise, you will realize that your flexibility is improving day by day and you are able to bend forward much easily. You can perform this exercise for 5 to 10 minutes a day.

### Half twist pose

The half twist is great for your back, kidneys and also your digestive system. When you perform this pose, you help your body eliminate waste with ease. If you have eaten too much and are not feeling well then performing this pose will immediately help you feel lighter and the food you ate will get digested easily. To perform this pose, start by sitting with your legs folded under you. Now release the left leg from under you and cross it over your right thigh. Now breathe in and twist your body to the right. Your right hand must go around your back and your left hand must embrace your left foot. Stay in the pose for a few minutes and release. Repeat on the other side. You can perform this exercise for 5 minutes daily and this time should include both sides.

### Tree pose

Tree pose is a very powerful pose and something that lord Shiva is said to have practiced regularly. To perform the tree pose, start by standing straight and having your hands by your side. Now lift your right leg and place it perpendicular to your left thigh. You can use your hands to lift up the foot and place it adjacent to your left thigh. Now release your hand, stand straight and lift both your hands above your head. Join your palms in the air. This pose is great to correct your posture and will help you maintain a strong spine.

### Boat pose

The boat pose is a unique pose and will help strengthen your core muscles. The idea is to look like a boat by performing this pose. So start by sitting on the floor and stretching your legs out. Now lift your legs into the air and bend forward as much as you can. You can grab the back of your thighs or simply stretch your hands past your thighs. Remain in this pose for a couple of seconds before releasing.

### *Plough pose*

The plough pose is a level 5-exercise and should only be performed by those that have practiced yoga for some time. It is important that you not rush into anything and do everything at a set pace. The plough pose is great for your shoulder, lower back and also your stomach. To perform this pose, start by sleeping on your back. Now lift your legs up in the air and create a 90-degree angle. Slowly lift up your lower back from the floor and use your palms to support it. Now keep pushing your legs backwards until your toes touch the floor behind your head. Remain in the pose for a couple of seconds before slowly pushing your feet back up again and returning to neutral position.

These form the various complementary yoga poses that you can try out with your Tibetan rites and avail good health.

# Tibetan Singing Bowls

Singing bowls are metal bowls that are used to accompany meditational practices. These bowls are said to have originated in china, where the bowls are rung like a gong to signify the start or end of meditation. These singing bowls are said to create a sound that helps in soothing the mind and body.

The structure of a singing bowl incorporates a bowl that is round and hollow with tall sides. A wooden or metal mallet accompanies it, which is used to sound to generate the sound with the help of the bowl. The bowl can be made of metal or wood or even plastic.

The mallet is used to hit on the rim of the bowl, which produces vibrations that travel inside the bowl and create a humming sound. Different sized bowls create different sounds and so, they are played in succession to create soothing music.

You can buy the bowls from an online store and use them during meditation to help you relax and reel in a sense of calm. The idea is to enter a deep state of relaxation just by hitting the singing bowl once. You don't have to keep playing it to feel relaxed and just the one hit will suffice. If you are feeling stressed out, then just hit the bowl once and you instantly feel relaxed. Just hit the bowl and close your eyes. Your mind will start travelling inwards and your conscious will unite with your subconscious.

The chakras inside your body will start to rotate harmonically and with each successive sound, they will begin to cleanse thoroughly and rotate at a uniform speed. So you can use this technique as a supplementary action to the other chakra cleansing rituals.

You need not buy an entire set and can settle for just one large bowl. They are available in all types of metals including copper, zinc and silver. If you are looking to buy a good quality one that will grow in value over time, then you can settle for a gold singing bowl. There are many who buy copper ones, clean it, fill it with water, hit it with the mallet and then consume the water to cleanse their internal body.

For those interested in using the bowls the right way, there are online videos available that give exact lessons on how to use them to create proper healing music.

# Important Natural Supplements That Fight Inflammation

The Tibetans believe that good health is the key to a successful and happy life. The best way to do this is by maintaining a sound mind and a great physical body. The former can be attained by performing the meditation and the latter by performing the Tibetan rites. But despite these, many times, the body can fall prey to illnesses and so, it is important to strengthen the immunity of the body. The best way to do so is by consuming natural herbs that are rich in anti oxidants and help prevent internal inflammation.

Inflammation refers to the swelling of organs or any other part of the body. When an infection takes place, the body reacts by swelling. This inflammation is to be curbed to avail fast relief from the illness. This best way to prevent these inflammations is by consuming natural supplements regularly. These supplements need to be administered as the foods we eat lack proper nutrition and don't give our bodies the nutrition that it needs.

### Ginseng

Ginseng is an herb that has been used in Chinese medicine for hundreds of years. The herb contains several properties that help fight away illnesses and also strengthen the immune system. Ginseng contains ginsenosides, which affects the inflammatory cells and curbs them to the highest possible extent. So those looking to better their immunity can consume this herb. It is available in both tablet and powder form, which can be bought online. It can also be bought whole, powdered and added to boiling water to prepare ginseng tea.

### Gingko Biloba

Gingko Biloba is another herb that is said to help increase immunity. Just like Ginseng, this herb contains anti-inflammatory properties that make it ideal to be consumed and the person can easily improve his or her immunity. This supplement can be availed in tablet or powder form and consumed.

### Noni

Noni is a unique fruit that is pre dominantly grown in Asia. This fruit is rich in anti oxidants and is often referred to as the elixir to life. The fruit is pressed and its medicinal properties are distilled in the form of a syrup which when consumed regularly can help reduce the effects of free radicles in the body.

### Vitamin c

Vitamin c supplements are essential when it comes to increasing the immunity in your body. Although consuming foods rich in the nutrient like oranges and lemons is a good choice, it is also important to consume a supplement, which contains vitamin c. you can avail vitamin c tablets or capsules and consume them on a regular basis. If you are unable to find it in your drugstore then look for it online. Similarly, it is also important to consume vitamin D supplements, as it will help in the absorption of calcium, which is required to build strong bones and teeth and maintain over all good health.

### Zinc

Zinc has both anti-inflammatory and cancer fighting properties and is an essential part of the human body. You can consume zinc rich foods such as mussels and other seafood or also opt for a zinc supplement. The dosage will depend on how zinc is already present in your body and you will have to ask your physician to prescribe the right dose for you.

### Fish oils

Fish oils as we know, are full of omega 3 fatty acids. Fatty acids are of two main types namely omega 3 and mega 6. Omega 6 fatty acids are bad for your heart and overall health whereas omega 3 is great for you. So to increase the amount of omega 3 fatty acids in your diet, you can incorporate fish oils. These oils have amazing anti-inflammatory properties and will allow your body to remain fit and healthy for a long time. Look for cod liver oil tablets or buy it in the oil form and consume one or two teaspoons full on a daily basis to improve your immunity and keep common coughs and cold at bay.

## Ginger

Ginger is a root that is known to help people remain healthy for a long time. Ginger is pound up and added to curries and teas as it will help in digestion and also prevent the onset of an infection. Ginger powder is also available, which can be added by the spoonful to curries or dissolved in hot water and consumed. You can add in a tablespoon full of palm sugar if you desire, as it will help in increasing the effects of ginger. Although many people peel the root before using it, it is best to leave the skin on as it contains a majority of the medicinal properties.

## Turmeric

Turmeric is also a root like ginger or rather a rhizome. Turmeric is rich in curcumin, which is a chemical that has cancer-fighting properties. It also has anti-inflammatory properties, which makes it ideal for fighting away infections. Most Asian cuisines add powdered turmeric to their curries and you can do the same. You can also grate some fresh turmeric, mix it into a glass of warm milk and consume it at night before retiring to bed and avail a good night's sleep.

Green tea

Green tea is the most preferred anti oxidant rich drink in the world. Its anti inflammatory properties makes it an over all winner. Although drinking green tea twice or thrice a day is the best solution, you must also consume green tea supplements, which will help you, increase your immunity. You can look for the supplements online or at a drug store.

These form the various supplements and their uses and you can consume them to remain healthy and strong. But don't over do anything in a bid to turn healthy faster. Allow your body to adjust to one supplement before moving to another.

# The 5 Rites And Food Rules

As we know, colonel Bradford completely immersed himself in the 5 rites and made sure that everything that deals with it is exploited to the fullest. This included knowing about the foods that can be eaten and those that are not permitted. These foods are regular foods, as the monks did not have access to any fancy and modern foods. So it is important for you to follow these food rules as well, if you make the most of your 5 rites routine.

Colonel Bradford understood from the monk's diet that, they did not mix two or more major nutrients, which could easily clash inside their digestive system. This means, if they were to consume proteins and carbohydrates together, then neither would be digested properly. So the rule of thumb was to consume one major type of nutrient and not confuse the body. So if you are to consume bread, then consume bread alone and don't mix it up with something filled with proteins like lentils. And if your bread is giving you carbohydrates then supplement it with more carbohydrate rich foods such as potatoes.

If you don't pay attention to this small aspect and continue consuming foods that can clash with each other, then your body will start to experience all sorts of difficulties including indigestion, flatulence and bloating. You will also have to push harder for the 5 rites to work on your body and it will impact you negatively.

So it is important to not have the food groups mixed up and maintain only a single nutrient type. Your body will digest all the foods effectively and you will be left with a lot of energy to conduct your day-to-day activities.

Now I understand that it will be tough for you to make dietary changes, especially if you are already accustomed to a steady diet. You might feel like it is a big task for you to change up your meals and watch what you are eating. But it is something that needs to be done, if you want to experience better health. You need not rush to make these changes and can take it slow. If you make one change per week, then it will not have a big impact on your body and it will have all the time in the world to adjust.

The best thing to do is to separate your starchy foods such as breads and rice along with fruits and vegetables away from your meats and lentils as also your fish and eggs. So these different categories of nutrients will not mix with each other and they will be separate.

The next rule to follow is to chew your food down completely. In this day and age, people don't chew their food for even the minimum required time. Chewing or masticating food is extremely important, as all the nutrients should be broken down inside your mouth. So this chewed food will pass down to your liver and gut and make it easier for these to digest the food. If you simply swallow the food, then these two organs will have to work over time to digest the food. It will take time for the complex nutrients to break down and in the process; the toxins present in food will not be broken down and eliminated from the body. The monks would chew the food for at least 30 minutes and not rush their eating. So make sure you eat for 20 minutes at least and don't rush it.

One big rule that most monks try to incorporate into their diet includes consuming egg yolks. Yes that is correct, raw egg yolks, as they are full of proteins. These proteins are important for your body and you need to incorporate it into your diet as much as possible. This egg yolk needs to be consumed either before a meal or after a meal. It should never be part of your diet. You can have 2 or 3 and the best thing is to have them fresh. So don't separate them in the morning and try to separate them just when you are about to consume them. Don't worry if you are a vegetarian as eggs are allowed for vegetarians. But if you really are averse to consuming eggs then skip this step. Don't forcibly eat something that your body does not want you to.

As a general rule, it is always better to consume 5 to 6 small meals as opposed to the standard 3 big meals. The body will have the chance to break down the nutrients in a better way. If you give it big meals then not all the food will properly be broken down and it will put a lot of pressure on the liver. So split your 3 meals in such a way that they turn into 3 small meals. But remember that you are only splitting them and not have 6 regular sized meals.

For all those interested in aging at a slower pace, It is best to start by eating all the right foods, which will not just help you remain youthful on the outside, but also on the inside. One of the main ways to do that is by consuming foods that are good for the body as a whole. So incorporating those ingredients that are full of anti oxidants is a great way to improve your looks. All you have to do is look for green vegetables and green tea and red fruits and regular tea. All of these are loaded with anti oxidants and will help your skin remain youthful and elastic.

One main rule to follow is to always eat your meals at the same time every day. If you start changing it up then your body will start over producing the acid in your body. If at any time there is acid secretion and no food in your stomach, then this acid will not only corrode the lining of your stomach but also get mixed with the blood and start circulating inside your body. So it is important to cut down on the amount of acid in your body and eat neutralizing foods.

There is a list available on the Internet that tells you which foods are acidic and which are not. You must consume the foods that are not acidic and cut down on the acid inside your body. There is a diet that caters to this form and you can look into it and adopt it to cut down on the acid content.

The Tibetan monks grow their own vegetables and you can do so too! You can plant them and harvest them and use them for all your food preparations. You don't need a big pile and can be self-sufficient. See how much your family eats and grow accordingly. Once you have harvested enough, you can also preserve them to last you a long time. You can make use of any preservation technique including drying, freezing, dehydrating and canning. This form of self-sufficiency will go a long way in helping you save on your costs and it will also be a sustainable way to get your hands on organic fruits and vegetables.

Apart from these, you already read about the various other foods related criteria that you need to bear in mind if you want the 5 rites to work for you. These, food needs, go hand in hand with the exercises and so does a healthy mind. It is best for you to entertain only positive thoughts and not give into the negative ones. Although it is known that a weak body will promote a weak mind, it can also be the other way round. So your weak minds can enable a weak body. So make sure you are trying your best to remain mentally positive and helping your body remain strong.

# How To Make It A Habit

It is important to make these exercises a regular habit and in fact, turn them into your lifestyle. For that, you have to follow a set pattern of rules, which are mentioned as under.

### *Research*

Remember that research is everything when it comes to alternate sciences. These are not things that you have grown up learning and need to start from scratch on them. For this, you have to read as much as you can on the subject and educate yourself thoroughly. Don't stop at this book alone and read as much as you can from as many sources as possible. Don't allow any spurious material to cloud your thinking and make sure that you are forming the right opinion on the matter. You can also join a group that discusses and practices the fiver rites of Tibetan and learn new benefits of these five rights.

## Schedule

Create and follow a regular schedule for these rites. If you don't have a schedule, then you will end up missing out on performing them. Don't affect this schedule in any way and find yourself the right time and place to perform these. Don't think someone will judge you and carry on with your rites even if you have on lookers. Make sure you reach the spot on time on a daily basis and this can include your balcony or your terrace. The air needs to be crisp and fresh and morning times are the best to carry out these rituals.

## Company

You can always ask someone to join you and have company when you perform these rituals. These can be your friends or your family members or even your neighbors. Having just one other partner with you is always rewarding for both of you. If any one of you is being lazy and not performing then the other can encourage you and vice versa. But respect their limits and don't force them to do it if they are not readily interested in performing the activities. Remain as devoted as possible and make the most of your opportunities.

## Record

Maintain a consistent record of all your activities. This will ensure that you remain motivated and know how much progress you are making. Don't give up on it at any time at all, as your body would have attained a momentum. You must keep supplementing this momentum and continue practicing these rites. Write down how much you weighed at the beginning of the practice and how much you weigh now. The drastic change in weight will help you continue with your exercise routines and allow you to experience a new level of confidence that is supplemented with good health.

## *Reward*

It is wise to reward yourself from time to time. This reward need not always be monetary and can be something that you really love and crave for. This includes buying yourself some nice clothes or shoes or even a day at the spa or an entire day for shopping. A nice fancy meal once in a while is also a great treat. Just make sure you don't indulge in rewarding yourself too often as it can turn into a habit and cause you to get accustomed to it.

These form the various ways in which you can turn the 5 rites into a lifestyle change.

# Conclusion

A visit to the Himalayas may perhaps be a distant and farfetched dream for many of us. But it is possible to incorporate some peace and some tranquility into our hectic lives. It is definitely possible to experience a slice of the Himalayas every day. We can transport ourselves mentally to the Himalayas and experience a state of bliss by following these movements. These Tibetan rites energize us and help us cope with the challenges of our daily lives with equanimity. Simply invest 10 minutes and 5 simple steps for unlimited energy and restored health. You're worth it!

If you enjoyed this book, please take the time to share it with your friends and post a positive review on Amazon. I would greatly appreciate it!

# RECOMMENDED READING

TANTRIC SEX: Couples Guide: Communication, Sex And
Healing
hyperurl.co/tantric


Tantric Massage: For Couples: Essential Guide To Love
Making & Couples Massage
hyperurl.co/tantricmas

# You May Enjoy My Other Books

Below you'll find some of my other popular books on Amazon. You can also visit my author page.

hyperurl.co/MarySolomon

HEARING GOD'S VOICE FOR BEGINNERS

smarturl.it/heargod

HEALING : Heal Your Mind, Heal Your Body: Change Your Life

hyperurl.co/selfhealing

AFFIRMATIONS and ASCENDED MASTERS: Achieve A Higher Consciousness

hyperurl.co/affirmations

CRYSTAL HEALING ENERGY

smarturl.it/crystala

CHAKRA HEALING EXPOSED

smarturl.it/chakraaa

Printed in Great Britain
by Amazon